PRACTICAL CLINICAL MEDICINE
Series Editors J. Fry and G. Sandler

W0050406

STROKES

C. Warlow, D. Wade, P. Sandercock, J. Muir, A. House, J. Bamford, R. Anderson and C. Allen

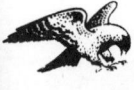 **MTP PRESS LIMITED**
a member of the KLUWER ACADEMIC PUBLISHERS GROUP
LANCASTER / BOSTON / THE HAGUE / DORDRECHT

Published in the UK and Europe by
MTP Press Limited
Falcon House
Lancaster, England

British Library Cataloguing in Publication Data

Warlow, Charles
    Strokes.—(Practical clinical medicine
    series)
    1. Cerebrovascular disease
    I. Title   II. Series
    616.8′1   RC388.5

ISBN-13: 978-0-85200-831-7   e-ISBN-13: 978-94-011-7724-5

DOI: 10.1007/ 978-94-011-7724-5

Published in the USA by
MTP Press
A division of Kluwer Academic Publishers
101 Philip Drive
Norwell, MA 02061, USA

Library of Congress Cataloging in Publication Data

Strokes.

    (Practical clinical medicine)
    Includes index.
    1. Cerebrovascular disease.   I. Warlow, Charles,
1934–   II. Series.   [DNLM: 1. Cerebrovascular
Disorders.   WL 355 S9215]
RC388.5.S857   1986   616.8′1   86-27552

Typeset and printed by Butler & Tanner Ltd, Frome and London

STROKES

CONTENTS

LIST OF AUTHORS

Dr Chris Allen,
Neurology Department,
Addenbrooke's Hospital,
Hills Road,
Cambridge

Mr Robert Anderson,
Institute for Social Studies
   in Medical Care,
14 South Hill Park,
London

Dr John Bamford,
Neurology Department,
The Radcliffe Infirmary,
Oxford

Dr Allan House,
University Department of
   Clinical Neurology,
The Radcliffe Infirmary,
Oxford

Dr John Muir,
General Practice Health
   Maintenance Study,
The Radcliffe Infirmary,
Oxford, and
The Surgery,
Woburn, Bedfordshire

Dr Peter Sandercock,
Neurology Department,
The Walton Hospital,
Rice Lane,
Liverpool

Dr Derick Wade,
Rivermead Rehabilitation
   Hospital,
Abingdon Road,
Oxford

Dr Charles Warlow,
University Department of
   Clinical Neurology,
The Radcliffe Infirmary,
Oxford

Series Editors' Foreword

Backing up the pioneering medical researchers and experimenters are the phalanxes and cohorts of practising clinicians in district general hospitals and in general practice who may have to implement and apply any breakthroughs and advances in practical and realistic terms. This they cannot, and should not, be expected to do without careful consideration and analysis. It is essential, therefore, to have regular reviews of the growing points of medicine which are constructively critical as well as being enthusiastic and which can present the issues and implications clearly and fairly to clinicians.

The *Practical Clinical Medicine* series is designed to provide such regular reviews on selected subjects. Each volume is under the charge of an invited editor who selects his team of 4–6 experts. Each contribution is an authoritative, detailed and referenced examination of his topic, is clearly presented in an understandable manner and is practical, relevant and applicable to everyday clinical practice.

The series is intended as a means of communication between researchers and practising clinicians. It is dedicated to generalists who provide primary health care in general practice and to generalists providing secondary medical care in district

general hospitals. Both are involved in applying good general
practical clinical medicine for their patients, but can only
succeed in a climate of constant review and examination.

JOHN FRY
GERALD SANDLER

ACKNOWLEDGEMENTS

Most multiauthor books identify the authorship of each chapter. This one does not, because we have written the whole thing together. How was that possible? Firstly, because we have all worked together in various combinations over the years and have tried to exchange ideas, criticisms and our own individual bits of expertise for the benefit of our patients with stroke, and to enhance our research efforts into stroke. In writing this book each of us wrote the first draft of one or two chapters and then read all the chapters, commented on them, changed them and gradually hammered the whole thing into shape.

We have attempted to see the problem of stroke from the general practitioners' perspective and indeed one of us is a GP, and two of us are married to GPs. We all subscribe to the view that the dichotomy between 'hospital care' and 'community care' has gone too far, and that for patients with stroke and their carers this system often works against them; a stroke *service* may have to be based in a hospital, but it must reach out into the community and work with the primary health care teams.

We are indebted to the many general practitioners and consultants who have allowed us to study their patients in Oxford, Bristol, and London, and indeed to the patients themselves and their families. We would like to thank our busy and underpaid secretaries who typed the manuscript and the various organizations which have supported our research, and us, at various times; the Medical Research Council, the DHSS,

ICI Pharmaceuticals, the Special Trustees of Guy's Hospital, and the Chest, Heart and Stroke Association.

CHARLES WARLOW
DERICK WADE
PETER SANDERCOCK
JOHN MUIR
ALLAN HOUSE
JOHN BAMFORD
ROBERT ANDERSON
CHRIS ALLEN

1

THE EPIDEMIOLOGY OF STROKE AND TRANSIENT ISCHAEMIC ATTACK

It is sometimes suggested that the results of epidemiological studies, whilst providing broad and general information, are not particularly relevant to individual patients. Although this chapter necessarily will deal with broad groups of patients rather than individuals, it is the study of such groups which allows not just the size of the problem to be identified, but also potential risk factors for strokes to be recognized which, in many instances, can then be modified in the individual patient. Fundamental problems in epidemiology are the introduction of bias by studying highly selected groups of patients (e.g. only those admitted to hospital) and small numbers, leading to uncertain estimates of the truth. Despite their relative frequency compared with many other conditions, the number of patients with stroke in any individual practice is small, yet the factors which may influence the characteristics of a practice population are legion and to a large extent impossible to quantify. Therefore the purpose of this chapter is to provide sufficient information about the incidence of, and risk factors for, stroke and transient ischaemic attack (TIA) in the community as a whole, to allow practitioners to relate this to their own individual patients.

DEFINITIONS

The term stroke will be used throughout this book since we agree with others that 'stroke is a consequence of a long term process and not a chance or random event as the term cerebrovascular accident (CVA) implies'. At the outset it is important to define clearly what type of patients are being discussed since the diagnostic labels of stroke, and more especially CVA, are often used extremely loosely.

For practical purposes a clinical definition of stroke is required, yet it must be able to use any additional information derived from the various investigations which may be performed. The following points should be included:

1. symptoms should develop rapidly and, with the exception of cases of subarachnoid haemorrhage, should reflect a *focal* disturbance of cerebral function;
2. the symptoms should have no apparent cause other than that of vascular origin;
3. the symptoms should last more than 24 hours or lead to death.

Investigations, such as a CT scan, may increase the certainty that the symptoms have an underlying vascular cause (see Chapter 4). The term 'vascular origin' is used to exclude patients with, for example, intracranial haemorrhage following head trauma or haemorrhage into a cerebral tumour.

The persistence of symptoms for more than 24 hours is the only part of the definition which distinguishes cases of stroke from cases of transient ischaemic attack (TIA). The division is arbitrary, and in practice most TIA only last a matter of minutes or hours. The philosophy behind the division is similar to that distinguishing angina from myocardial infarction – the assumption is made that TIA are due to ischaemia which is so short-lasting that brain function recovers quickly and completely, whilst strokes are due to cerebral infarction and more or less irreversible damage to the brain. Some authors make a further division by time into major or minor stroke (the latter is sometimes referred to as a reversible ischaemic neurological deficit or RIND). The terms minor stroke and RIND suggest that the patient has made a complete recovery in a matter of weeks, and this division may be of value in identifying a subgroup of stroke patients with a better prognosis. It must be emphasized that some symptoms which are common in general practice, such as dizziness, vertigo, and syncope, are not considered as focal neurological disturbances (see Chapter 3).

TYPES OF STROKE

Stroke is no more than a descriptive term for the end-point of several different pathological processes, in the same way that anaemia is the common end-point of many disorders of haemopoiesis. Nobody would now consider grouping together patients with macrocytic anaemia due to vitamin B_{12} deficiency and those with microcytic anaemia due to menorrhagia. The necessity of separating patients according to underlying pathological processes is clear. It is due to the difficulties of distinguishing different pathological types of stroke (as will be discussed in Chapter 4) that this logical approach is often not applied in clinical practice and is one explanation of the divergent findings of different research studies. Therefore, if we are to advance our understanding of risk factors, potential treatments and outcome, we must consider groups of stroke patients that are as homogeneous as possible.

The first step towards this goal is to consider separately those patients with the well recognized underlying processes of *cerebral infarction* (*CI*), *primary intracerebral haemorrhage* (*PICH*) and *subarachnoid haemorrhage* (*SAH*). Data from the

Oxfordshire Community Stroke Project (OCSP), where the underlying process has been confirmed in a very high proportion of patients, show that about 80% of cases of first ever stroke are due to CI, 9% to PICH and 6% to SAH (there were also 5% of cases where the stroke type was uncertain). It seems likely that, in current UK practice, fewer than 70% of patients with acute stroke are admitted to hospital. Whilst the characteristics of patients who are admitted and those who remain in the community differ in ways that are difficult to describe accurately, it is known that hospital-based series, which are prominent in the stroke literature, tend to contain an excess number of cases of PICH (because they tend to be more serious) and miss a proportion of mild ischaemic strokes (because the patients stay at home). The implications of such selection bias to GPs dealing with patients in the community are clear, and suitable caution should be employed when interpreting the results of hospital-based studies of stroke.

INCIDENCE

There are many studies of stroke incidence and a conspicuous feature has been the wide variation in the reported rates. Various hypotheses have been proposed to explain this variation but critical evaluation of the methodology of these studies should come first. The most reliable data are likely to come from prospective, community-based studies. Stroke has a relatively low case fatality rate and so the analysis of death certificate diagnoses is not an accurate method of measuring incidence, and the enormous limitations of retrospective case note review are well known. One must also be very clear which strokes are being counted – for studying incidence and natural history it is important that only patients having their *first-ever* stroke are included.

Some standardization is achieved by relating the findings of an individual study to a reference population with a known age and sex structure, such as that of England and Wales.

Using this method the overall incidence of first-ever stroke is about two per 1000 persons per year. If recurrent strokes are included the rate is about 25% higher. However, age- and sex-specific rates are of considerably more value, and those for first-ever stroke in Oxfordshire are shown in Figure 1.1. Not only do they allow individual practitioners to calculate the likely number of strokes in their practice, given its age and sex structure, but they clearly demonstrate that the majority of patients are over 65 years of age. Amongst those patients aged greater than 85 years the rates approach 20 per 1000 persons per year. On average, a GP will see four or five new cases of stroke every year.

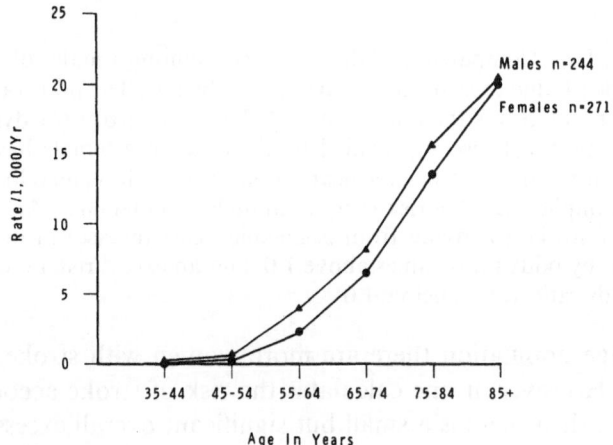

Figure 1.1 The age- and sex-specific incidence of first-ever stroke in Oxfordshire. Data from 515 patients in the Oxfordshire Community Stroke Project (1981–4)

The incidence of TIA has been less well studied. It is impossible to know how many patients never come to medical attention, because of the transient nature of the symptoms. A minimum estimate from the Oxfordshire Community Stroke Project is about 0.5 per 1000 persons per year. In other words, a GP is likely to see one or two new cases every year.

The greater life expectancy of women means that in the

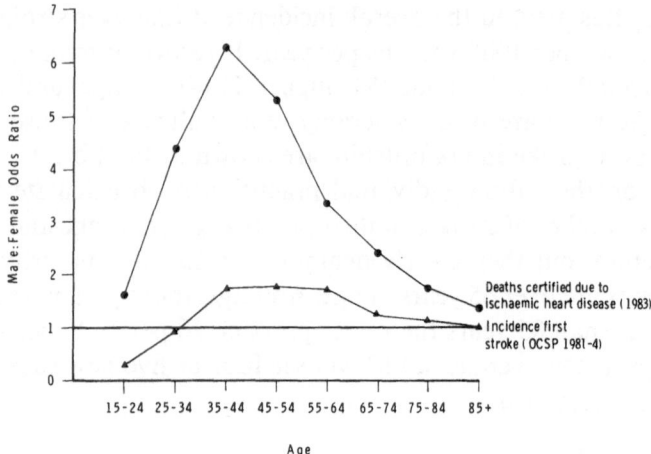

Figure 1.2 Comparison of the excess risk amongst males of stroke with death due to ischaemic heart disease by age. The odds ratio on the vertical axis is the odds of a male having a stroke (or dying of ischaemic heart disease) divided by the odds of a female having a stroke (or dying of ischaemic heart disease). Therefore, an odds ratio of 1.0 implies that the risk is equal in males and females. An excess risk of stroke (or dying from ischaemic heart disease) in males is shown by odds ratio values above 1.0, and an excess risk in females by odds ratio values below 1.0

average population there are more women with stroke than men. However, if one calculates the risk of stroke according to sex, then there is a small but significant overall excess risk amongst men. In Oxfordshire this is about 30%, and similar figures have been reported from most Western countries. The pattern of male excess risk with age is similar, though less marked, to that of deaths due to coronary heart disease with the greatest excess being between the ages of 45 and 64 years (Figure 1.2). It has been suggested that this sex difference is due to some protective hormonal factor in women which is lost after the menopause.

Figure 1.3 shows that the incidence of *all* types of stroke increases with age. This even applies to SAH, which is not a disease confined to the young as some reports from neuro-surgical centres might have led one to believe.

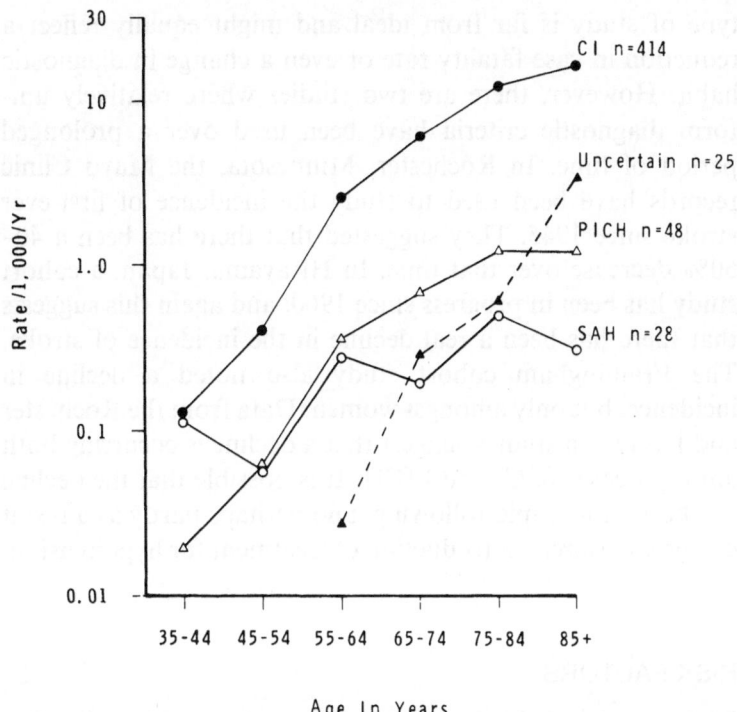

Figure 1.3 The incidence of first-ever stroke by stroke type. Data from the Oxfordshire Community Stroke Project (1981–4). Note the logarithmic scale

Prevalence

Most estimates of stroke prevalence (i.e. the total number in a community on a particular day) are calculated from incidence rates and survival data. In this way the estimated prevalence of stroke is between five and ten per 1000 persons at any one point in time.

Trends in incidence

Studies of death certification first suggested that the incidence of stroke might be declining although, as noted above, this type of study is far from ideal and might equally reflect a reduction in case fatality rate or even a change in diagnostic habit. However, there are two studies where relatively uniform diagnostic criteria have been used over a prolonged period of time. In Rochester, Minnesota, the Mayo Clinic records have been used to study the incidence of first-ever stroke since 1945. They suggested that there has been a 40–50% decrease over that time. In Hisayama, Japan, a cohort study has been in progress since 1960, and again this suggests that there has been a real decline in the incidence of stroke. The Framingham cohort study also noted a decline in incidence, but only amongst women. Data from the Rochester and Hisayama studies suggest that a decline is occurring both amongst cases of CI and PICH. It is possible that the decline has been more rapid following, and perhaps partly as a result of, the widespread introduction of treatment for hypertension.

RISK FACTORS

Risk can be defined as 'the chance of sustaining a bad outcome', and therefore one can determine the risk of stroke for a whole range of factors in the population. Of course, a positive correlation will be found not only when the factor has a pathogenetic link with the development of stroke, but also when the factor is itself the result and not the cause of a common underlying disease. Long lists of associations are not particularly useful to the individual practitioner, who will be most interested in those potentially alterable factors which have a direct pathogenetic link with the development of stroke, particularly those which enable patients most at risk of developing stroke to be identified. This section will concentrate on such factors.

Risk can be described in three different ways, each of which provides somewhat different information. The *relative risk* of stroke compares the frequency of a particular characteristic (e.g. diabetes) amongst patients with stroke and amongst an age- and sex-matched, stroke-free population. This is used to identify potential factors which may increase the likelihood of stroke. If a group of patients with a characteristic are followed to see how many develop stroke, then the *absolute risk* for that characteristic, i.e. the rate at which such patients develop stroke, can be determined. Obviously this is useful when assessing an individual patient. From the point of view of large-scale preventive medicine, it is important to know the *attributable risk* – that is, the proportion of all strokes which might be accounted for by the characteristic, which is a reflection of both the absolute risk and the prevalence of that characteristic in the community. Thus, a characteristic with a high absolute or relative risk of stroke, but with a low prevalence (such as atrial fibrillation associated with rheumatic heart disease), may have a lower attributable risk (and thus a lesser public health importance) than a characteristic which carries a lower absolute risk of stroke but is very common (e.g. raised blood pressure). There are far fewer studies which describe absolute and attributable risks than relative risk, yet it is the former which are of more direct importance to practitioners who are trying to prevent stroke.

Factors linked to the pathogenesis of stroke

Blood pressure

One can make a case for abolishing the word 'hypertension', which makes the false assumption that there is some valid dichotomy between 'hypertension' and 'normotension'. An association between severely raised blood pressure and stroke (in particular PICH) has been recognized for many years, but it is likely that the attributable risk of long-term but quite modest elevations of blood pressure due to the promotion of atherosclerosis and cerebral infarction is considerably greater. It is prudent to consider blood pressure amongst middle-aged people and the elderly separately, as the prevalence of coexisting disease and likely treatment options differ.

It has been shown repeatedly that the higher the level of

systolic or diastolic pressure when measured in middle age, the higher the risk of *all* forms of stroke subsequently, with the possible exception of SAH. Two points from the Framingham study are worth emphasizing. Firstly, the gradient of increasing risk is steeper for increasing systolic pressure than for diastolic pressure, and indeed isolated raised systolic pressure is a risk factor *irrespective* of the diastolic pressure. Patients with systolic blood pressures above 180 mmHg have about an eight times greater risk of stroke than patients with systolic blood pressures below 120 mmHg. However, the Framingham study was unable to show any 'safe' lower limit. The implications of this fact for stroke prevention will be discussed in chapter 10.

In the elderly the situation is more complex, mainly because of the frequent presence of other factors, such as cardiac disease, which independently increase the risk of stroke but which also tend to lower the blood pressure. Some cross-sectional studies have suggested that both systolic and diastolic blood pressure increase with age up to the sixth decade, following which there may be a decline. This pattern, however, has not been borne out in longitudinal studies. Isolated raised systolic blood pressure is more common in the elderly, and was present amongst 11% of the Framingham cohort aged 70–79 years. Although this is often dismissed as a reflection of the rigidity of the arterial wall, in Framingham the increased risk of stroke with raised systolic blood pressure continued at least until the age of 75, and appeared to be present even if indirect measurements of arterial wall rigidity were taken into account. The Framingham authors concluded that the use of diastolic blood pressure in the elderly might be positively misleading.

There is a large amount of evidence which links raised blood pressure and stroke, the overall relative risk being about six. The importance of this factor, however, lies in the high prevalence of the condition; perhaps four million people in the UK have diastolic blood pressures between 100 and 120 mmHg, i.e. there is a high attributable risk.

Lipids

Raised serum cholesterol has been strongly linked with the development of coronary heart disease, yet its relationship with stroke, and in particular cerebral infarction, is much less clear. However, if total cholesterol levels are considered, the relationship even with coronary artery disease is much less marked over the age of 55 years, although the relationship continues if subfractions of cholesterol are considered – i.e. a positive relationship for low-density lipoprotein (LDL) cholesterol and a negative relationship with high-density lipoprotein (HDL) cholesterol. The Framingham study showed a modest negative relationship with HDL cholesterol and cerebral infarction in both sexes. Amongst women, however, there was also a substantial *negative* relationship with LDL cholesterol despite a positive correlation for coronary artery disease in the same cohort. A similar finding was reported from Hawaii. This apparent difference between cerebral infarction and coronary artery disease is puzzling and requires further investigation. It also emphasizes the quantitative, and sometimes even qualitative, differences between the risk factors for myocardial infarction and cerebral infarction.

Acute myocardial infarction (MI)

This must be distinguished from merely a distant history of MI, because both embolism from left ventricular mural thrombus and hypotension may be the cause of stroke in the context of acute MI. Detailed information is lacking, but it seems that less than 2% of acute MIs are complicated by stroke. An even lower proportion of strokes are due to acute MI.

Atrial fibrillation (AF)

Considerable caution is needed when interpreting data relating to AF. In the past many cases of AF were due to rheumatic heart disease when the dilated left atrium frequently contained thrombus which could embolize to the brain. In Framingham the relative risk of stroke in this situation was 17. However, with the decline of rheumatic heart disease a much higher proportion of cases of AF are now due to ischaemic heart disease. In this situation the relative risk of stroke is about six, which is only of about the same magnitude as the relative risk of left ventricular hypertrophy as seen on the ECG. One cannot assume that there is always a pathogenetic link between AF and stroke in an individual patient; the AF may only be a marker for generalized atheromatous disease in the coronary as well as the cerebral arteries.

Diabetes

The association between diabetes and vascular disease is well recognized. Prospective studies such as that in Framingham have shown that it has its greatest impact on peripheral vascular disease. However, it is clear that the presence of diabetes increases the relative risk of stroke two to three times, and may have an attributable risk of about 10%.

Haematocrit

Patients with polycythaemia rubra vera have an excess risk of thromboembolic events, including cerebral infarction. Patients with a 'high normal' haematocrit (45–50%) probably only have a modest excess risk of cerebral infarction, particularly when the frequently associated features of hypertension and cigarette smoking are taken into account.

Smoking

An independent effect of smoking can be demonstrated, particularly amongst men, but the association is weak compared with that in coronary artery disease and seems to be confined to men under the age of 65.

Oral contraceptives (OC)

Whilst there does seem to be an excess risk of stroke amongst women who have used the combined OC pill, one must be aware of the undesirable but understandable tendency for unexplained strokes amongst such women to be ascribed to its use. Also, much of the data relate to the era of relatively high oestrogen dose pills. It is thought that the relative risk of stroke with OC use is about three but the absolute risk is very low (perhaps 1 in 10 000 OC users per annum) and the population attributable risk is minute.

Alcohol

Studies from Finland have suggested that there is an association between 'binge' drinking, as practised in that country, and stroke. This is perhaps related to dehydration or to an effect on blood pressure. No convincing evidence has been reported to link chronic alcohol ingestion with an increased risk of stroke independently of other associated conditions such as raised blood pressure, smoking and cardiac disease.

Markers of vascular disease

Although they are often described as risk factors for stroke, the conditions described below represent other manifestations of degenerative vascular disease. The frequency with which stroke occurs amongst patients with these conditions can be determined, and may be useful when considering primary prevention of stroke.

Transient ischaemic attacks

The natural history of TIA will be described in chapter 5. Their transient nature means that estimating their frequency retrospectively is difficult; however, perhaps 20% of patients with stroke have had at least one preceding TIA. The risk of developing a stroke following a TIA is about 5% per annum.

Asymptomatic carotid bruit

The presence of a localized bruit over the carotid bifurcation is usually a sign of greater than 40% stenosis of the underlying vessel, and is thus a useful marker of vascular disease. Over the age of 65 years, up to 5% of the population may have a carotid bruit. However, a totally occluded artery does not produce a bruit while stenosis of the external carotid artery does. Carotid bruits are not just a sign of carotid disease but are also a strong indicator of *generalized* vascular disease in other arteries. The stroke rate is about 2% per annum but half of these will be in the contralateral hemisphere. Overall, the relative risk of stroke is about two, which is the same as the relative risk for myocardial infarction in the presence of a carotid bruit.

Cardiac disease

Whilst acute myocardial infarction and atrial fibrillation may have a pathogenetic link with stroke in some individuals (but certainly not all), there are other manifestations of cardiac disease which have been associated with stroke. These include angina, any past history of MI, congestive heart failure, left ventricular hypertrophy defined by ECG criteria, and cardiomegaly seen radiographically. These are all associated with hypertension; therefore one would expect the risk of stroke to be increased. However, the Framingham study has shown that these conditions increase the risk of stroke independently of hypertension. The relative risk of stroke is three times higher in patients with coronary artery disease and five times higher if the patient is in overt heart failure or has ECG evidence of left ventricular hypertrophy.

Stroke risk profile

Everyday experience shows that many of the conditions described frequently coexist, and that many are highly prevalent in stroke patients. The 323 patients in the Oxfordshire Community Stroke Project who were seen in 1981–3 with a first-ever stroke had the risk factors shown in Table 1.1.

Table 1.1

Hypertension*	53%
Angina and/or past myocardial infarction	32%
Peripheral vascular disease	23%
Transient ischaemic attacks	20%
Atrial fibrillation	14%
Cervical arterial bruit	12%
Diabetes mellitus	9%

*Blood pressure greater than 160/90 on two or more occasions *before* the stroke.

The interaction between these factors is not well documented though various investigations have attempted to produce stroke risk profiles. In Framingham, nearly 50% of the strokes could be predicted from only 10% of the asymptomatic population using a combination of systolic blood pressure, glucose intolerance, serum cholesterol, cigarette smoking and ECG left ventricular hypertrophy. However, it is clear that, with the exception of age, raised blood pressure is the single most important risk factor for stroke.

PRACTICAL POINTS

Epidemiology provides a framework derived from *populations*, which helps to decide the management of *individual* patients. Although stroke is a common disease, an average general practitioner will see only four or five new cases every year. There are several easily recognizable disorders which, if present in an individual, increase the risk of stroke; particularly high blood pressure, any kind of cardiac disease, diabetes mellitus, transient ischaemic attacks, and a localized arterial bruit in the neck.

Most stroke patients have one or more obvious risk factors at the time of the stroke, and often these risk factors have been obvious for years. A summary of the definite and possible risk factors for cerebral infarction, primary intracerebral haemorrhage and subarachnoid haemorrhage is given in Tables 1.2–1.4.

Table 1.2   Risk factors for cerebral infarction

Definite	Possible
Increasing age	Increasing blood cholesterol
Male sex	Increasing plasma fibrinogen
Increasing blood pressure	High normal haematocrit
Cardiac disease	Smoking
myocardial infarction	Increasing obesity
angina	Excess alcohol consumption
atrial fibrillation	Peripheral vascular disease
cardiac failure	
cardiomegaly	
left ventricular hypertrophy	
Diabetes mellitus	
Cervical arterial bruit	
Transient ischaemic attack	
Oral contraceptives	
Polycythaemia rubra vera	

Specific treatments are available for many of these factors but whether stroke risk is reduced depends on there being a cause and effect relationship.

Table 1.3   Risk factors for primary intracerebral haemorrhage

Definite	Possible
Increasing age	Oral contraceptives
Increasing blood pressure	Excess alcohol consumption
Anticoagulation	
Coagulation disorders (e.g. hae-mophilia)	

Table 1.4   Risk factors for subarachnoid haemorrhage

Definite	Possible
Increasing age	Increasing blood pressure
Female sex	Oral contraceptives
Anticoagulants	Excess alcohol consumption
Coagulation disorders (e.g. hae-mophilia)	

THE CAUSES OF STROKE AND TRANSIENT ISCHAEMIC ATTACKS

Atheromatous disease in the arteries supplying the brain causes about 80% or more of all transient ischaemic attacks (TIA) and strokes due to cerebral infarction; emboli from the heart, blood disorders and non-atheromatous arterial diseases account for the remainder. Hypertension is the main cause of primary intracerebral haemorrhage, and the rupture of an intracranial aneurysm or arteriovenous malformation (AVM) are the commonest causes of subarachnoid haemorrhage. Most of the important treatable causes of stroke can be identified from the history, a physical examination and a few simple investigations.

STROKE AND TIA DUE TO CEREBRAL INFARCTION

Atheromatous arterial disease in large arteries

Atheromatous disease of the large arteries supplying the brain can produce cerebral ischaemia or infarction by a variety of

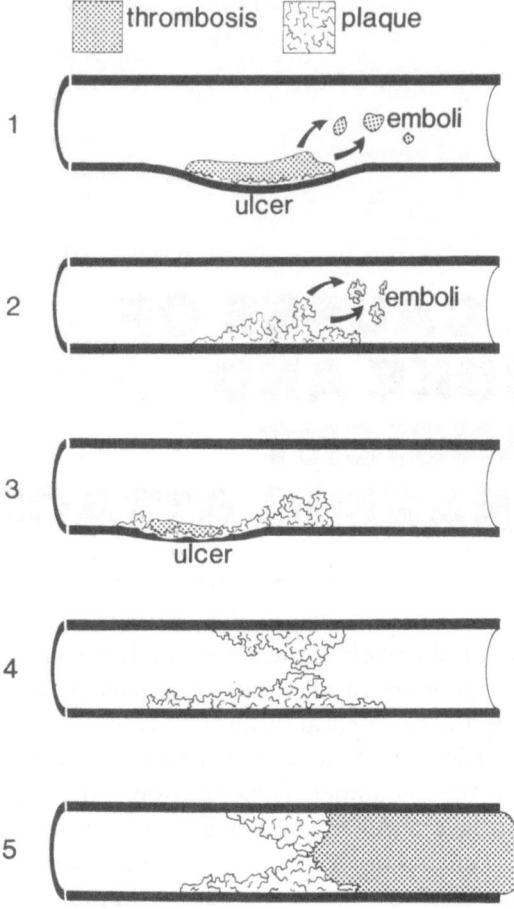

Figure 2.1 The different stages of atheromatous disease in the internal carotid artery and the various ways they may cause TIA and cerebral infarction.

1. Ulceration: platelet-fibrin thrombus forms on the base of an atheromatous ulcer and then parts break off, sending emboli distally.
2. Plaque disruption: debris, such as bits of cholesterol or fibrous tissue, can break off and embolize. Lipid material, which is very thrombogenic and may cause vessel occlusion, is released if a plaque fissures.
3. Complex lesion: ulceration, plaque disruption and thrombus formation may all occur simultaneously.

mechanisms (Figure 2.1). Whether infarction actually occurs depends on how long an artery is occluded for, the collateral blood supply beyond the occlusion, and by how much the local cerebral blood flow is reduced.

Figure 2.2 shows the commonest sites for atheroma in the arteries to the brain.

Hypertension is one of the most important factors which accelerates the rate of formation of plaques, and also makes them develop more distally in the arteries supplying the brain. The relationship between hypertension and the interactions between flowing blood and the atheromatous plaque that lead to thrombosis, embolization or occlusion is less clear.

Disease of the small vessels in the brain

Hypertension not only accelerates the formation of atheroma in the neck arteries, but also leads to progressive disorganization of the small arteries perforating the deep brain substance, notably in the basal ganglia and brain stem. Occlusion of these small arteries may give rise to 'lacunar infarction' (see Chapter 4) while their rupture causes the typical hypertensive haemorrhages within the basal ganglia.

---

4. Reduction of flow (so-called haemodynamic TIA or cerebral infarct). When stenosis is very severe (greater than 80%), flow may be reduced at times of relatively mild hypotension and cause ischaemia or infarction (e.g. the sort of drop in BP associated with standing up, a cardiac arrhythmia, a heavy meal or starting vasodilator treatment). This mechanism of stroke and TIA is rare.
5. Occlusion: plaque fissure or build-up of surface thrombus may lead to occlusion. However, if the collateral supply through the circle of Willis or other channels is adequate, occlusion of even the internal carotid artery can occur without causing any symptoms at all

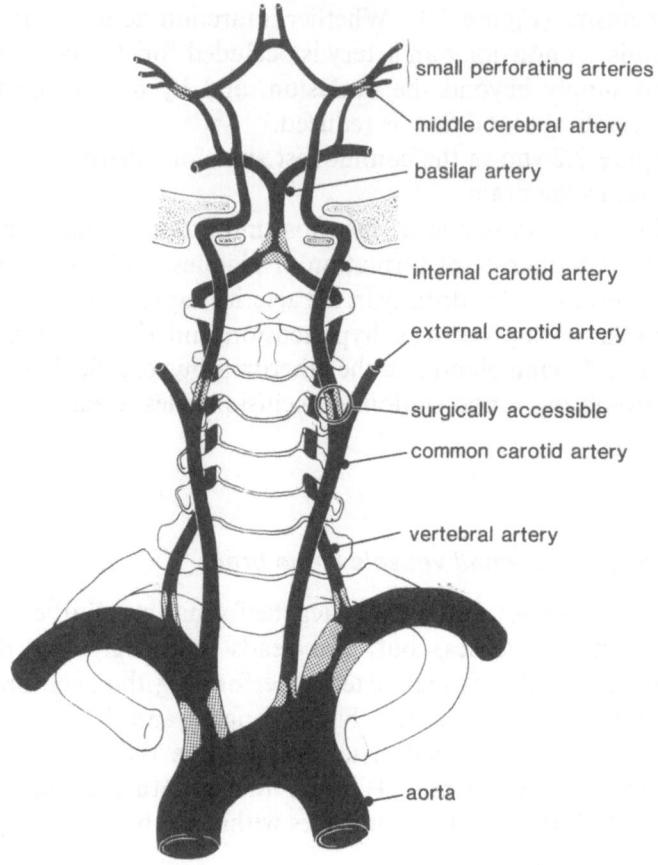

small perforating arteries

middle cerebral artery

basilar artery

internal carotid artery

external carotid artery

surgically accessible

common carotid artery

vertebral artery

aorta

Figure 2.2 The sites of atheroma in the arteries supplying the brain. The commonest site is the origin of the internal carotid artery. This is the only site easily accessible to surgery and endarterectomy

Clinical diagnosis of atheromatous arterial diseases

It is wise to try and make a positive diagnosis of atheroma as the cause of TIA or cerebral infarction for two main reasons. Paradoxically, the most important is that non-atheromatous arterial diseases such as arteritis or dissection may require urgent treatment. Secondly, patients with TIA and minor ischaemic stroke due to atheromatous lesions of the internal carotid might possibly be suitable for carotid endarterectomy (see Chapter 5). Table 2.1 gives the factors that increase the chance of such a lesion being present. However, as Figure 2.3 shows, the presence of a bruit does not always indicate atheroma, and conversely the absence of a bruit does not rule out the possibility. A small ulcer or plaque big enough to cause emboli may not cause a bruit (Figure 2.3, nos. 3 and 4):

> A 65-year-old man suddenly developed numbness and weakness of the left face and arm. The symptoms resolved completely within 2 weeks. He had smoked 20 cigarettes a day for many years, had been on a diuretic for hypertension for 2 years, and had a myocardial infarction 10 years ago. No carotid bruit could be heard. CT scan was normal. An angiogram showed an ulcerated plaque at the origin of the right internal carotid artery (Figure 2.4). The stroke was probably due to cerebral infarction as a result of embolism from the carotid plaque, and the risk of recurrent stroke might be reduced by carotid endarterectomy (see Chapter 5).

Table 2.1 Factors which point towards atheroma as the underlying cause of cerebral infarction

History of	Examination
Age greater than 40	Bruit over carotid artery (see Figures 2.3 and 3.1)
Intermittent claudication	
Hypertension	Bruits over other arteries (e.g. femoral)
Diabetes	
Ischaemic heart disease	Absent pulses in legs and feet
Hyperlipidaemia	Blood pressure difference between right and left arms (generally a sign of subclavian stenosis or occlusion)
	Xanthelasma

Non-atheromatous arterial diseases

These are all rare causes of stroke and are outlined in Table 2.2. In most cases the patient will have few or no risk factors for, or clinical evidence of, atheromatous arterial disease else-

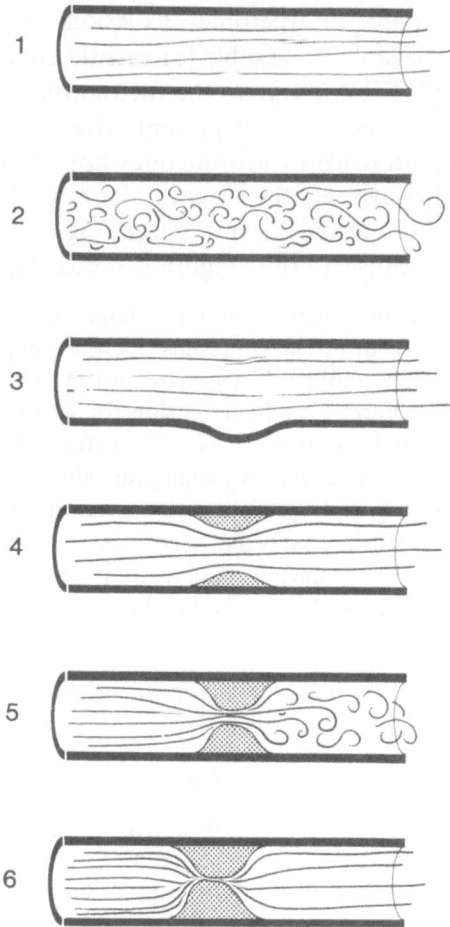

Figure 2.3 Carotid bruits and their relationship with arterial lesions
likely to cause TIA or cerebral infarction.

Lesion	Risk*	Flow	Bruit
1 None	No	Laminar	No
2 None	No	Turbulent†	Yes
3 Ulcer	Yes	Laminar	No
4 Small plaque	Yes	Laminar	Perhaps
5 Large plaque	Yes	Turbulent	Yes
6 Tight stenosis	Yes	Minimal	No

* Risk of TIA and cerebral infarction

† For example, high cardiac output (anaemia, thyrotoxicosis, intracranial
arteriovenous malformation) or aortic stenosis

Table 2.2 Non-atheromatous arterial diseases

	Clinical clues
Inflammatory arterial disease	
Giant cell arteritis	Systemic illness
	Headache
	Weight loss
	Malaise
	Joint stiffness/myalgia
Systemic lupus erythematosus	Systemic illness
	Already known to have SLE
	Young stroke (age < 40)
	Rash, arthropathy, renal disease
	Raynaud's phenomenon
Polyarteritis nodosa	Systemic illness
	Purpuric rash
	Livedo reticularis
	Lung or renal disease
	Eosinophilia
Non-inflammatory arterial diseases	
Non-penetrating arterial injury	Blow to neck
	Sudden neck extension (e.g. Yoga, strangulation, whiplash injury)
Migraine	Onset of stroke during typical migraine attack
	Gradual evolution of symptoms
Syphilis	History of contact
	Homosexual
Oral contraceptives	
Extreme rarities (e.g. fibromuscular dysplasia, homocystinuria, drug abuse	Young stroke

where. There may well be clinical clues such as systemic illness or a raised ESR to point to arteritis, for example. Hospital referral for a complete assessment is generally wise if one suspects non-atheromatous arterial disease.

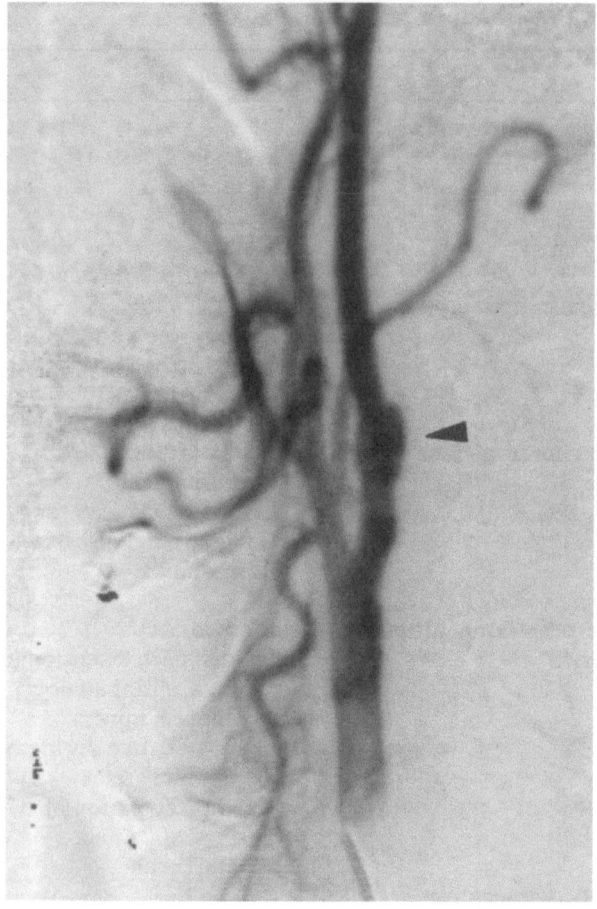

Figure 2.4 Carotid angiogram showing an atheromatous ulcer (black arrow) at the origin of the internal carotid artery

Arteritis

Giant cell arteritis must be confirmed by biopsy (Chapter 6).

A 70-year-old lady had an episode of blurred vision in the right eye lasting an hour. She had been unwell for the past month, not eating well, complaining of stiff shoulders and she said that she had avoided combing her hair because it made her scalp sore. The ESR was 50. Temporal artery biopsy showed giant cell arteritis.

The clues were all there. She had no vascular risk factors other than her age. The duration of her visual loss was much longer than the brief visual loss of amaurosis fugax due to atheromatous thromboembolism (which usually lasts seconds or a few minutes at most) and the constitutional upset and symptoms of polmyalgia pointed to giant cell arteritis. Visual loss in this context warrants immediate treatment with high-dose steroids (80 mg daily of prednisolone) until the biopsy result is available.

Migraine

Some ischaemic strokes undoubtedly begin during a typical migraine attack, though quite what migraine is, and whether it causes the cerebral infarction, is open to debate. Just occasionally a 'migrainous stroke' can be the first manifestation of classical migraine:

> A 50-year-old scientist noted a blank spot in the centre of vision in both eyes. He could read words around the blank spots at first, though he realized a few minutes later that the words no longer made sense. Fifteen minutes later, when he tried to speak to his secretary, the 'words came out all jumbled up'. His speech returned a few minutes later. He felt unwell and drove home. In the car, tingling and numbness gradually spread up over his right arm and on to his face and he then developed a severe unilateral headache. The numbness persisted for 48 hours. He had never had migraine in the past. A CT scan was normal. He subsequently had several attacks of classical migraine.

The sedate evolution of one neurological deficit into another (in this case central scotoma, followed by dyslexia, then dysphasia and finally cortical motor/sensory problems) is highly characteristic of migraine.

Arterial injury

Internal carotid dissection may require urgent treatment with anticoagulants to prevent the thrombus that forms on the torn intima occluding the vessel, and certainly requires diagnosis if there is any likelihood of legal action:

A 20-year-old football fan developed a mild right hemiparesis on the way home from the pub one Saturday night. He was a non-smoker, normotensive with no evidence of cardiac disease. Angiography showed a tapering left internal carotid artery occlusion typical of dissection (Figure 2.5). His hemiparesis resolved as a result of, or despite, anticoagulant treatment. He later admitted

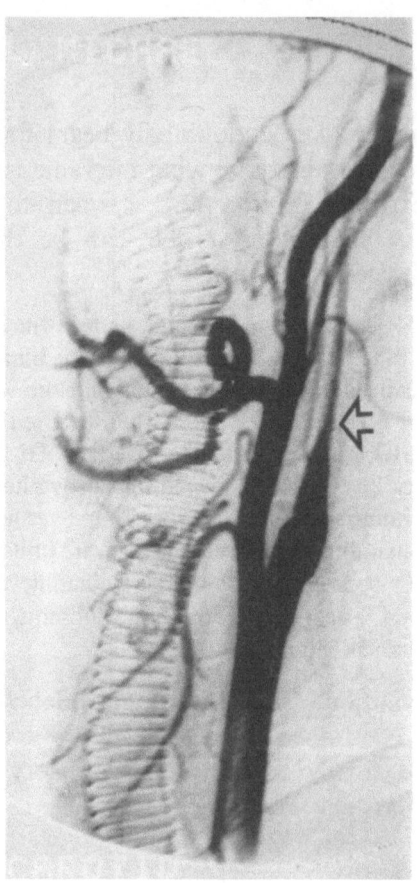

Figure 2.5 Carotid angiogram showing a tapering occlusion of the internal carotid artery (open arrow) resulting from dissection induced by being grabbed round the neck in a fight

that he had been held around the neck in a post-match fight in the pub, a neck-stretching injury which was presumably sufficient to tear the intima and start the arterial dissection.

Embolism from the heart to the brain

A wide variety of cardiac lesions can release emboli consisting of different materials into the cerebral circulation: fibrin, platelets, cholesterol, calcium and infective vegetations. Not all of these emboli, such as the calcified debris from a calcific and stenosed aortic valve, can be prevented by giving either anticoagulants or antiplatelet agents. Cardiac sources of embolism include (numbers on the list indicate key to Figure 2.6):

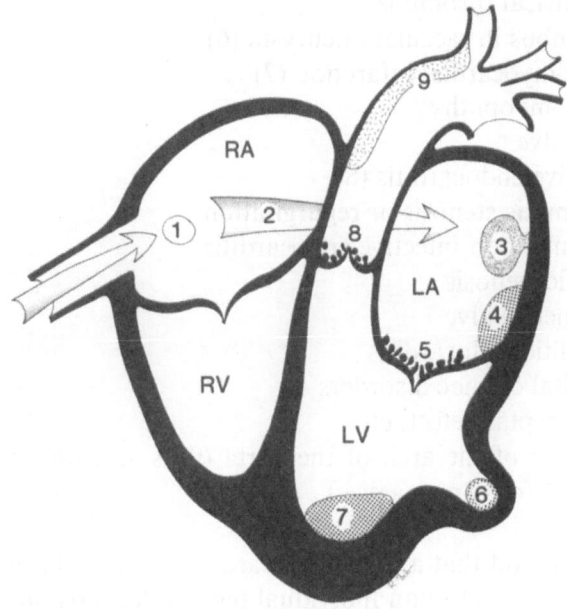

Figure 2.6 Some of the cardiac lesions which can release emboli into the circulation. See text for key

Left atrium
  Paradoxical embolism from the venous system (1) passing
  through a patent foramen ovale (2)
  Myxoma (rare) (3)
  Left atrial thrombus due to atrial fibrillation (4)
  Sinoatrial disease
Mitral valve
  Infective endocarditis (5)
  Rheumatic stenosis or regurgitation
  Marantic non-infective endocarditis
  Mitral annulus calcification
  Mitral leaflet prolapse
  Prosthetic valve
Left ventrical thrombus
  Thrombus in saccular aneurysm (6)
  Acute myocardial infarction (7)
  Cardiomyopathy
Aortic valve
  Infective endocarditis (8)
  Rheumatic stenosis or regurgitation
  Marantic non-infective endocarditis
  Calcific stenosis
  Prosthetic valve
  Syphilitic endocarditis
Congenital cardiac disorders
  Atrial septal defect, etc.
(Dissection of the arch of the aorta (9) is also illustrated in
Figure 2.6 for convenience.)

The likelihood that a particular cardiac lesion is the cause of
a cerebral infarct in an individual patient depends on several
factors. For example, in patients with atrial fibrillation the
risk of having a stroke is increased threefold if rheumatic heart
disease is present as well. Stroke in these circumstances occurs
because thrombus forms in the left atrium and then breaks up,
causing embolization to the brain and elsewhere. On the other
hand, in elderly patients the presence of atrial fibrillation may

just be a marker of generalized vascular disease affecting both the heart and the brain; in other words the cerebral infarct is not necessarily due to emboli from the heart, but perhaps to arterial disease in the neck. The problem is that in an individual patient it can be almost impossible to be certain of the mechanism of the stroke:

> A previously fit 80-year-old lady suddenly developed a left homonymous hemianopia. She had been in atrial fibrillation for the past 10 years, but had no evidence of rheumatic heart disease. Her systolic blood pressure had varied between 180 and 200 mmHg for years. The cause of the stroke was very difficult to sort out: it could have been a cerebral infarct due to embolism from the heart or to hypertensive small vessel disease within the brain. It could also have been a small primary intracerebral haemorrhage (about 15% of patients with primary intracerebral haemorrhage are in atrial fibrillation).

Blood disorders causing TIA and cerebral infarction

These are all rare causes of strokes and are listed below. They can be identified by simple blood tests:

Red cells	Polycythaemia rubra vera
	Secondary polycythaemia
	Sickle cell disease
	Severe anaemia
	Paroxysmal nocturnal haemo-globinuria
White cells	Leukaemia
Platelets	Essential thrombocythaemia
Proteins	Paraproteinaemias

PRIMARY INTRACEREBRAL AND SPONTANEOUS SUBARACHNOID HAEMORRHAGE

These are relatively uncommon, but are nonetheless very important since urgent surgical treatment may be required for cerebellar haemorrhage and subarachnoid haemorrhage (see Chapters 4 and 6). Table 2.3 shows the commonest causes.

The following history emphasizes the need to think of sub-arachnoid haemorrhage in anyone with a *sudden* onset of headache (or neckache); the headache need not necessarily be all that severe.

Table 2.3   Causes of intracranial haemorrhage

Causes of intracerebral haemorrhage
Hypertension
Blood disorders (see below)
Arteritis
Amyloid angiopathy (this type *only* affects the brain)

Causes of subarachnoid haemorrhage
Intracranial aneurysm
Arteriovenous malformations
Mycotic aneurysm (associated with infective endocarditis)
Blood disorders (see below)

Blood disorders causing intracranial haemorrhage (all rare causes)

Red cells	Aplastic anaemia
White cells	Leukaemia
Platelets	Thrombocytopaenia
Coagulation factors	Warfarin overdosage
	Haemophilia

A 16-year-old girl returned to the newsagent after her newsround. As she got off her bike she said she felt ill, and vomited on the pavement. She was taken inside the shop and complained of neckache. Her father collected her and took her home. She told the GP she felt ill with headache, neckache and backache. The GP's initial diagnosis was 'flu. She later became drowsy and was admitted to hospital with a provisional diagnosis of viral meningitis. Lumbar puncture and CT scan (Figure 2.7) both con-firmed subarachnoid haemorrhage, and cerebral angiography showed a small posterior communicating artery aneurysm which was successfully clipped.

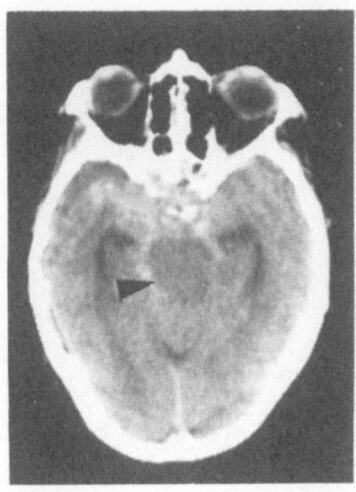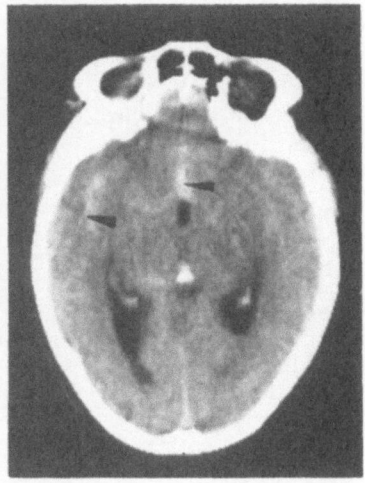

Figure 2.7 CT scan showing blood (white, high-density areas arrowed) in the subarachnoid space, around the brainstem (left panel), in the interhemispheric fissure and in the left Sylvian fissure (right panel)

PRACTICAL POINTS

Atheromatous disease of the arteries supplying the brain is the commonest cause of cerebral infarction and TIA.

The probability of finding atheromatous disease in the cerebral arteries is increased if the patient is aged over 40 and has risk factors for vascular disease, or has vascular disease elsewhere (e.g. angina, claudication).

Carotid bruits are a useful, but not infallible, guide to the presence of an atheromatous lesion at the carotid bifurcation.

A cardiac lesion in a patient with a TIA or cerebral infarct is not always the cause of the event. Furthermore, some patients with a cardiac lesion may turn out to have stroke due to primary intracerebral haemorrhage.

Non-atheromatous arterial diseases can usually be diagnosed by simple bedside assessment and an ESR.

3

THE DIAGNOSIS OF TRANSIENT ISCHAEMIC ATTACKS

A transient ischaemic attack (TIA) is defined in clinical terms: an acute loss of focal brain or ocular function with symptoms lasting less than 24 hours and which, after adequate investigation, is presumed to be due to embolic or thrombotic vascular disease. The 24-hour distinction between TIA and stroke is arbitrary; it is likely that focal ischaemic episodes which last minutes, hours or several days have similar causes, should be investigated in the same way, have more or less the same natural history, and require identical treatment. The main difference is that short attacks (lasting minutes) are more often recurrent than longer attacks (lasting days).

TIAs are common. About 25 000 people with a TIA consult their doctor every year in the United Kingdom for the first time, so that an average general practitioner sees about one or two new cases every year. In addition, he will see the same number, or more, who might have had a TIA but in fact have something else requiring completely different management. Indeed, many of the conditions which masquerade as TIA are far easier to treat than the ravages and complications of atheromatous vascular disease. Because the diagnosis of TIA is essentially 'clinical' and so often has to be based on a good history after the attack, and because they are not so common that they are easy to diagnose, there can be difficulty getting the diagnosis right both for the general practitioner, and for the hospital specialist. Getting it right matters not so much for the patient who really has a TIA (for whom the bottom line of treatment is the control of vascular risk factors which could and should be done whenever the patient consults the doctor), but for the patient who has something else which may require specific and effective treatment, or just plain reassurance, rather than inappropriate use of aspirin or other apparently simple remedies.

MAKING THE DIAGNOSIS OF TIA VERSUS NOT-TIA

To make the diagnosis of TIA the following seven questions must be answered 'yes':

Was the attack focal rather than non-focal?
Has migraine been excluded?
Has epilepsy been excluded?
Have 'psychogenic' attacks been excluded?
Have peripheral nerve lesions been excluded?
Has hypoglycaemia been excluded?
Have structural lesions of the brain or eye been excluded?

Focal versus non-focal attacks

Occlusion of an artery to the brain or eye (by thrombosis, embolism, trauma, inflammation, etc.) almost always causes *focal* loss of function rather than non-focal or global symptoms. Focal symptoms include:

monocular visual loss (whole field, or part of one field) i.e. amaurosis fugax;
unilateral weakness (arm, leg, face in various combinations);

unilateral numbness, deadness, pins and needles (arm, leg, face in various combinations);
language disturbance (aphasia, alexia, agraphia);
homonymous hemianopia;
dysarthria;
diplopia;
dysphagia.

Non-focal symptoms are almost always due to a general reduction in cerebral blood flow, and are more likely to be caused by a drop in systemic blood pressure than occlusion of a cerebral artery. Given this distinction it is clear that the causes include cardiac arrhythmias, postural hypotension, vasovagal syncope, and acute vasodilation (as a result of drugs, after meals, etc.). Non-focal symptoms are characterized by a sudden feeling of faintness, bilateral dimming or loss of vision, generalized weakness, buzzing in the ears, sounds becoming distant, generalized prickling and sweating, and loss of consciousness. Such symptoms *may* occasionally occur during a TIA but there are always prominent focal symptoms as well.

Rotational vertigo as an *isolated* symptom is not generally regarded as a TIA, although it can occur during brainstem ischaemia, because other causes are probably much more common, e.g. labyrinthitis, positional vertigo, Menière's disease. Simultaneous bilateral weakness or sensory disturbance can also occur in a brainstem TIA but is very easily confused with functional overbreathing (see below) unless accompanied by more overt brainstem symptoms (e.g. dysarthria, diplopia).

Non-focal symptoms are often due to highly treatable conditions and must not be labelled as TIA so giving a completely false sense that everything possible that can be done is being done, and even that the prognosis is worse than it really is:

Mr Stokes, a 70-year-old, had three episodes of sudden loss of consciousness without any warning. He was referred to a local physician. On examination there was a left carotid bruit and the ECG showed left bundle branch block. Aspirin was prescribed for the 'TIA' but, after two more attacks, he was seen by a neurologist who referred him at once to a cardiologist. A 24-hour ECG revealed periods of complete heart block, the aspirin was stopped, and a permanent pacemaker abolished his attacks. The carotid bruit was a red herring because the attacks were 'non-focal'; about 5% of asymptomatic 70-year-olds have carotid bruits.

Migraine

Common migraine should never be confused with a TIA, and nor should a typical attack of classical migraine consisting of a spreading and intensifying neurological aura (usually visual) lasting about 20 minutes and followed or accompanied by headache often in association with nausea and vomiting. Patients with classical migraine sometimes experience their very familiar aura but without the headache, and are usually delighted rather than worried that something other than migraine is happening to them. However, some people – at any age – can start having migrainous auras, without any headache, and they require reassurance that they are not about to have a stroke. The diagnosis is made entirely on the history and can be difficult. A migrainous aura develops and intensifies over several minutes, reaches a maximum in perhaps 5–10 minutes, and fades in perhaps 10–30 minutes. Often there are positive symptoms (flashing or zigzagging lights) rather than the negative symptoms of ischaemia (blindness, weakness) and the disturbance tends to spread from one cerebral function to another, e.g. speech is affected first and *then* vision, rather than both simultaneously. Perhaps the diagnosis of migraine without headache should always be confirmed by a neurologist.

Epilepsy

Two main seizure types can be confused with focal ischaemia. Firstly, sudden inability to speak – speech arrest – is probably more often epileptic than ischaemic, whereas clear-cut dysphasic speech with hesitations, word-finding problems, use of wrong words, or disordered grammar is much more likely to be ischaemic than epileptic. Secondly, sensory epilepsy, like focal ischaemia, tends to cause tingling, burning, or even pain but the symptoms 'march' across the hand (or foot) and up the limb and spread from one part of the body to another on the same side. Ischaemic symptoms tend to start in all of the affected parts simultaneously:

> A 65-year-old man presented with frequent attacks of tingling in the left hand, buttock, and trunk. These attacks did not affect each part simultaneously but spread from one to the other over about 30 seconds. He was started on aspirin for 'TIA'. After a few weeks the sensory symptoms were accompanied by jerking of the left hand and arm, by which time it was quite clear they were epileptic. A CT scan revealed a right parietal glioma and the plan to do a carotid angiogram for his 'TIA' was abandoned.

Psychogenic attacks

Overbreathing causes tingling around the mouth, in the fingers or in the toes, but is not necessarily accompanied by feelings of shortness of breath, or indeed of panic. Usually the patients are younger than the typical TIA patient and devoid of any strong risk factors for stroke. The attacks tend to be provoked by anxiety-inducing situations and can sometimes be precipitated by asking the patient to overbreathe in the surgery. Confusion certainly arises when, as sometimes happens, the tingling is *unilateral* rather than bilateral, and then the only clues to the diagnosis are the patient's age and the provoking situation. Hysterical weakness is not often transient and can usually be demonstrated on examination (sudden collapsing of the 'weak' part, unusual efforts and postures when making simple movements, inconsistencies in the weakness, etc.). Plain malingering can be difficult to sort out, and one tends to be slightly unsympathetic when it leads to inappropriate and unpleasant investigations like carotid angiography before the truth is revealed.

Peripheral nerve lesions

Pressure on peripheral nerves causes distal weakness and numbness, and has been experienced by everyone at some time. The context is usually obvious, e.g. waking at night, after leaning the elbow on a hard edge, etc. Indeed, many patients with genuine TIA try and write off their attacks as being due to this mechanism. However, after pressure on a peripheral nerve the numbness and weakness is always followed by *painful* pins and needles, which is unusual in a TIA.

Hypoglycaemia

Occasionally hypoglycaemia causes focal neurological symptoms, identical to those of a TIA, and without any general manifestations such as sweating, confusion and palpitations. Attacks tend to occur before meals or after exercise, and very particularly just after waking up in the morning. Almost always the patients are on hypoglycaemic drugs, though a very, very few turn out to have an insulinoma.

Structural lesions of the brain or eye

Transient focal neurological attacks can sometimes be a manifestation of brain lesions such as tumours, arteriovenous malformations, giant aneurysms, or subdural haematomas, but usually the symptoms are those of focal epilepsy rather than focal ischaemia. This cause of focal neurological attacks is extremely unusual. It is also a very rare presentation of these kinds of brain lesions.

Several ophthalmological disorders can and do cause transient monocular blindness, or the *symptom* known as amaurosis fugax:

ischaemia of the retina
papilloedema

glaucoma
migraine
retinal detachment
retinal haemorrhage
vitreous floaters
malignant hypertension
macular degeneration.

A 50-year-old lady was admitted under the vascular surgeons with several attacks of transient blurring of vision in one eye. Just before carotid angiography a neurologist was consulted, who pointed out the papilloedema and unilateral sensory neural deafness. A CT scan revealed an acoustic neuroma and obstructive hydrocephalus, and the patient was transferred to a more appropriate surgical service.

Ischaemic monocular blindness usually starts suddenly like a blind or shutter falling over the eye, or coming up from below; only the top or bottom half of the vision may be affected. The attack usually lasts a few minutes or less, there is no significant pain, and the retina itself is normal. During an attack emboli can sometimes be seen passing through the retinal circulation, but more commonly one can see small yellow sparkling cholesterol emboli impacted at arteriolar branching points since these tend to persist for days or weeks after the attack. If there is any doubt about a *local* cause for the symptoms (e.g. glaucoma) the patient must be seen by an ophthalmologist.

It is extremely important not to assume that every attack of focal neurological disturbance, particularly in the elderly, is necessarily due to ischaemia.

THE CAUSE OF THE TIA

Once the diagnosis of TIA, rather than something else, has been made, one has to consider whether the cause is embolism from the heart, a haematological disorder, a rare arterial disease, or – more than likely – the embolic or thrombotic complications of atheroma. This is not always easy to sort out.

Embolism from the heart

This should at least be suspected if:

a potential cardiac source of embolism is found (Chapter 2);
attacks have been in more than one arterial territory;
the patient is young (less than about 50);
no vascular risk factors;
no evidence of vascular disease (angina, claudication, vascular bruits).

The main difficulty is that potential cardiac sources of embolism *and* atheroma are common, particularly in the elderly, and knowing whether one or the other is *the* cause of a TIA can be completely impossible; this applies particularly to non-rheumatic atrial fibrillation. Given this difficulty it is probably best to confine management to the reversal of any vascular risk factors, and to treat the cardiac disease on its haemodynamic merits. Perhaps it is also reasonable to use a relatively safe antithrombotic drug such as aspirin (see Chapter 5).

Haematological causes of focal ischaemia

These are usually obvious if a full blood count and ESR are done, and also a sickling test in Negroes (see Chapter 2).

Non-atheromatous arterial diseases (Chapter 2)

Although rare, these are important, because there may be specific treatment (e.g. corticosteroids for giant cell arteritis) or a question of litigation (trauma to neck arteries). Vasculitic disorders usually declare themselves by generalized symptoms such as malaise or weight loss along with a high ESR, while trauma comes out in a good history of antecedent events such as a car crash, attempted strangulation, or a blow on the neck.

TIA caused by the complications of atheroma

This is in many ways a diagnosis of exclusion of the other causes of TIA, along with strong clues that the patient is the sort of person likely to have atheromatous disease. In other words he has one or more risk factors for stroke (see Chapter 1) or indeed for coronary artery disease:

increasing age
raised blood pressure
heart disease of any kind
localized cervical arterial bruits (see below)
diabetes mellitus
peripheral vascular disease
smoking
hypercholesterolaemia.

Not only is it important to identify risk factors as clues to the diagnosis, but they may require correcting (see Chapter 10). Often other vascular diseases require fairly intensive management as well (e.g. angina, claudication, uncontrolled atrial fibrillation, cardiac failure, aortic aneurysm, diabetes etc). TIA *can* occur in middle age, and *can* occur with no stroke risk factors, but this is distinctly unusual. However, one must be constantly aware of, and try and exclude, non-vascular causes of transient focal neurological events as well as non-atheromatous causes of TIA before jumping headlong into the inappropriate diagnosis of TIA due to atheromatous vascular disease, and then initiating a series of increasingly dangerous investigations and treatments.

Other conditions which may be due to transient ischaemia of the brain

Transient global amnesia

This is an unusual but very characteristic syndrome. A middle-aged or elderly patient rather suddenly develops severe anterograde amnesia which lasts for several hours. During this time, which is never subsequently recalled by the patient, no new information is retained for more than a few seconds and the same question is often asked repetitively. There is usually retrograde amnesia for months or years, but this recovers after the attack resolves. There are no other symptoms, and certainly no loss of personal identity. Some attacks are caused by ischaemia or epilepsy, but in the vast majority there is identifiable cause and the prognosis appears to be very good.

Drop attacks

Drop attacks tend to occur in middle-aged and elderly women. While walking, or occasionally just standing, the woman suddenly falls to the ground, usually badly bruising her knees or face. If there is any loss of consciousness it is only for a split second. Sometimes drop attacks are a manifestation of brainstem ischaemia but usually no cause can be found.

Subclavian steal

This is a very rare form of TIA which takes up a disproportionate amount of space in textbooks. There is stenosis or occlusion of a subclavian artery proximal to the origin of the vertebral artery which leads, during ipsilateral forearm exercise, to retrograde blood flow away from the brainstem down the vertebral artery into the arm. This usually causes no more than vertigo or a feeling of faintness.

Cervical spondylosis

This is very rarely a definite cause for focal brain ischaemia. Many elderly people feel 'dizzy' on looking up, but the exact cause of this symptom is not known. Clear-cut demonstration of vertebral artery occlusion during neck movement is extremely unusual.

INVESTIGATIONS

Investigations to establish the diagnosis of TIA, rather than something else, and to find the cause of the TIA, are largely self-evident if the above diagnostic strategy is followed. Routine investigations should include:

full blood count (?polycythaemia, leukaemia);
ESR (?vasculitis, myeloma, cardiac myxoma, bacterial endocarditis);
platelet count (?essential thrombocythaemia);
sickle-cell test in blacks;
urea and electrolytes if hypertensive or on a diuretic;
blood glucose (?diabetes);
syphilis serology;
cholesterol in young and middle-aged;
chest X-ray (?heart size, valvular calcification, enlarged left atrium);
ECG (?cardiac arrhythmia, left ventricular hypertrophy, ischaemic heart disease);
skull X-ray (?calcification of the carotid siphon, shift of the pineal).

Echocardiography

Echocardiography to delineate a structural cardiac cause of embolism to the brain or eye is only indicated if there is clinical evidence of this type of cardiac disease (symptoms, signs, chest X-ray, ECG) or if the patient is young and unlikely to have atheroma.

Twenty-four hour ECG monitoring

This procedure is fruitless unless the patient has had not a TIA but transient *non-focal* neurological attacks likely to be due to episodes of global reduction in cerebral blood flow caused by a cardiac arrhythmia.

Angiography

Angiography is required only if a policy of carotid endar-terectomy is being pursued (see Chapter 5). Angiography of at least the symptomatic artery should be done only if the patient has experienced a carotid distribution TIA (transient monocular visual loss, hemiparesis, hemisensory loss, language disturbance), is fit enough for surgery, and is willing to consider surgery. This is very much a question to be discussed after referral to a neurologist. The dangers of angiography are relatively small (about 2% risk of stroke or death) but the investigation requires hospital admission and is expensive, frightening and uncomfortable.

Many patients with TIA have localized arterial bruits in their neck (Figure 3.1) but this merely confirms vascular disease without specifying the exact vascular disorder. A carotid bruit is *not* necessarily an indication for carotid angiography, nor does it even mean that the patient has necessarily had a carotid TIA. About 5% of the elderly asymptomatic population have a carotid bruit. Moreover, the absence of a carotid bruit does *not* always mean that no arterial disease is present since an occluded or even very narrow artery may not cause a bruit at all (see Chapter 2).

CT scan

This will rule out most structural brain lesions causing, or masquerading as, TIA but this situation is so unusual that one

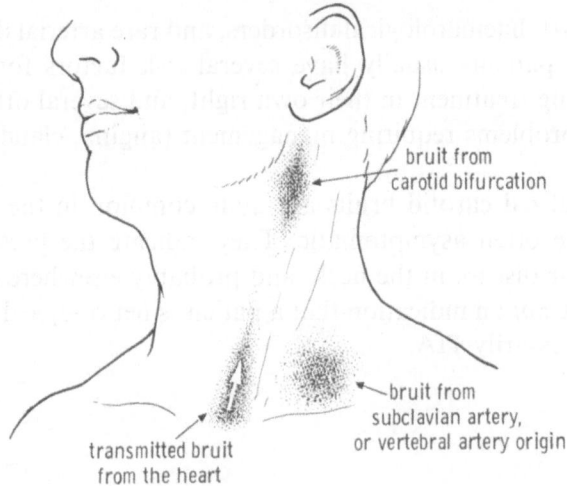

bruit from
carotid bifurcation

bruit from
subclavian artery,
or vertebral artery origin

transmitted bruit
from the heart

Figure 3.1 The typical sites of bruits in the neck arising from various sources. Reproduced from the *Oxford Textbook of Medicine* by courtesy of the Oxford University Press

could argue that the investigation is unnecessary, even if it were easily available. Certainly patients with monocular visual loss do not require it; nor probably do those with vertebrobasilar TIA.

PRACTICAL POINTS

Focal neurological attacks are not always TIA, even in elderly patients.

The diagnosis of a TIA depends on a careful history, and a few quite simple investigations which can be done by the general practitioner, or in outpatients.

Non-focal neurological symptoms (e.g. faintness) are almost always due to a sudden drop in blood pressure as a result of cardiac arrhythmia, postural hypotension, etc.

Most TIA are due to the embolic and thrombotic complications of atheroma, but some are due to embolism from the heart, haematological disorders, and rare arterial diseases.

TIA patients usually have several risk factors for stroke requiring treatment in their own right, and several other vascular problems requiring management (angina, claudication, etc.).

Localized carotid bruits are quite common in the elderly, and are often asymptomatic. They indicate the presence of vascular disease in the neck, and probably elsewhere as well, and are *not* an indication that a patient's neurological attacks are necessarily TIA.

4

THE DIAGNOSIS OF STROKE

There are four components to the diagnosis of a patient with a 'stroke':

1. Is it really a vascular problem?
2. What type of vascular lesion is present?
3. What is the cause of the vascular lesion?
4. What is the extent of the brain damage?

Firstly, the 'stroke' may be a manifestation of a mass lesion or some other non-vascular pathological process. If it is a stroke the next steps in diagnosis are to identify whether it is primarily ischaemic or haemorrhagic and then what the cause is. Finally, the extent of the damage should be established. The first three steps provide the information to institute acute treatment (Chapter 6) and secondary preventive measures (Chapter 11); the last helps determine the prognosis and plan rehabilitation (Chapter 7).

Simple clinical methods can provide the diagnosis of a vascular lesion (i.e. a stroke) and give an accurate estimate of the extent of the neurological damage. However, it is often impossible to diagnose the type and precise cause of the lesion. This is because in cerebrovascular disease, as in other disorders, several different pathological processes cause only a limited number of clinical syndromes. In the diagnosis of an individual with a stroke, it cannot be assumed that each pathology has its own unique combination of clinical features allowing it to be identified with complete accuracy.

CLINICAL PRESENTATION OF STROKE

The best known presentation of cerebrovascular disease is a sudden focal deficit of brain function which persists for more than 24 hours. The other well-known syndrome is due to subarachnoid haemorrhage (SAH) with an explosive onset of headache, vomiting and neck stiffness which may or may not be accompanied or followed by a focal deficit. However, vascular disorders of the brain do not always fit into such a tidy classification. There may be a more insidious onset of global loss of function (dementia and gait disturbance), occasionally a slowly progressive focal deficit, or epilepsy may be the sole presenting feature. Whilst a sudden focal brain lesion is very likely to be a stroke, just occasionally other pathological processes present in the same way. Dementia, a slowly progressive focal deficit, or epilepsy are more frequently manifestations of non-vascular lesions such as intracranial tumours. The diagnosic picture at the bedside is sometimes confused in individuals who have a mixture of several of these prime syndromes. So cerebral infarction may present with a slowly progressive hemiparesis with added episodes of acute weakness, and on examination there is dementia as well, and SAH may present with sudden headache and neck stiffness, at first with no focal signs, but some days later drowsiness and aphasia develop.

THE BEDSIDE DIAGNOSIS OF STROKE

Is it really a vascular lesion?

Many diseases can be misdiagnosed as a 'stroke' in a patient presenting with a hemiplegia, or other focal disturbance of brain function:

cerebral metastasis
malignant glioma, or meningioma
subdural haematoma
cerebral abscess
acute demyelination (multiple sclerosis)
post-ictal (Todd's) paresis
hypoglycaemic focal deficit
hysteria.

In the past, the risk of this mistake may have been as high as 10%, mainly because of a tendency to assume that every patient who presented with a hemiplegia had had a 'stroke'. However, with a careful history and examination the risk of being caught out should be substantially lower; less than 1%.

The presenting history

In a patient with an acute focal 'stroke' there are some clinical features which suggest an unsuspected mass lesion. Particularly careful attention should be directed to the nature and time course of the symptoms and the way in which the focal deficit evolved. In about one-third of patients an accurate history cannot be obtained from the patient because of aphasia, drowsiness or confusion. In this case it is always worth asking relatives or others (if necessary by telephone) about the patient's previous neurological state and the details of the event itself. If the neurological deficit really was sudden then almost always the activity being performed at onset is known (e.g. peeling potatoes, watching TV, etc.). Gradually progressive deficits can seldom be pinned down so precisely.

The absence of a clear history of sudden onset is grounds for suspicion that a non-vascular lesion is present, probably space-occupying in the head.

The evolution of the deficit

Most cerebrovascular lesions produce a deficit that reaches its maximal extent quickly, often within minutes and usually within hours. Such rapid evolution of a focal neurological deficit is unusual in non-vascular lesions. Later there may be some global deterioration (i.e. depression of conscious level) but the focal deficit is most often maximal at or near the onset. Sometimes gradual occlusion of an artery may produce a deficit which is slow to evolve, or does so in a stuttering fashion. Even then the focal deficit is usually complete within a day or two. 'Lacunar' strokes (see page 21), caused by the occlusion of fine perforating branches of the main cerebral arteries, often have a stuttering onset over days which may cause some diagnostic confusion with non-vascular lesions. However, the clinical deficits are recognizable as arising from a restricted volume of brain damage (see below) and are not accompanied by deterioration in conscious level, or evidence of raised intracranial pressure:

> A 56-year-old man, living alone, was seen because of a left hemi-plegia. He could only give a vague history that he woke 12 days before with weakness of his left side. This had initially improved but he had begun to fall repeatedly because of fluctuating left leg weakness. On the day the doctor was called by a neighbour the man complained that his left arm felt heavy, 'as if it doesn't belong to me', but the weakness of his leg was better. The GP found that he had a moderate hemiparesis, and marked visuo-spatial neglect. There was no papilloedema and he was fully alert. He was referred to hospital with the diagnosis of progressive carotid occlusion causing cerebral infarction. However, a CT scan showed a large malignant tumour in the depths of the right cerebral hemisphere with considerable cerebral oedema (Figure 4.1).

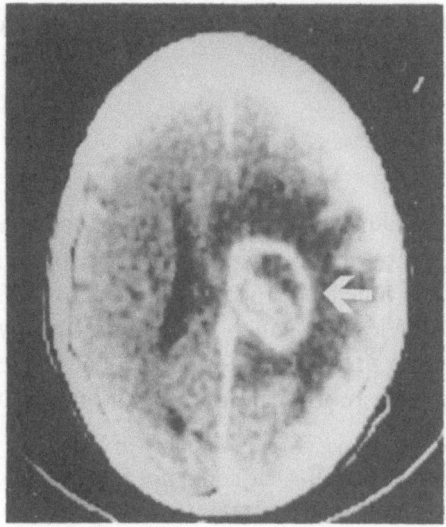

Figure 4.1 CT scan showing a malignant tumour (arrow) in the right cerebral hemisphere of a patient thought to have had a stroke

The lack of any clear history of a sudden onset in someone living alone was the cause of this diagnostic mistake (though referral to hospital was the correct management).

Cerebrovascular risk factors

Increasing age and evidence of extracranial vascular disease are common in stroke patients (Chapter 1). Some of the disorders which might be confused with stroke, such as multiple sclerosis, are much more likely to occur in younger people in whom stroke is very rare. Of course, heart disease and manifestations of atherosclerosis occur with increasing frequency with advancing age, so a middle-aged or elderly person with a non-vascular brain lesion may also (coincidentally) have some of these stroke risk factors. However, the complete absence of stroke risk factors should certainly arouse suspicion that a mass lesion is present. The younger and more generally 'healthy' a patient is, the more suspiciously should his doctor view an unexplained 'stroke'.

Epilepsy

Only 5% of patients with an acute stroke have a focal or generalized seizure at the onset (a larger proportion develop epilepsy at some time after the stroke, perhaps 10%). Most of the non-vascular lesions which can be confused with strokes are more likely to present with epilepsy. Therefore, the occurrence of seizures is another pointer to a non-vascular cause:

> A 65-year-old woman gave a distinct history that 3 days previously she had woken to find that she could not form her words properly. This had improved after 5–10 minutes but the next day she noticed some clumsiness of her right hand. She said that she had had no previous trouble but her relatives revealed that they had noticed her muddling up her words on occasions over the previous 3 weeks. On the day the woman called her doctor she had had a bout of twitching of the right side of her face for 5 minutes. Whilst the GP was examining her he saw a second attack which was a focal seizure affecting the right face and hand. On examination there was a left carotid bruit and a mild paresis of the right upper limb. The patient had some word-finding difficulties and the right plantar response was extensor. The GP referred the woman to hospital, quite reasonably thinking (because of the bruit) that she had critical stenosis of her carotid artery. Investigation showed that the patient had a malignant tumour in the left frontal region.

The carotid bruit was a red herring and occurs in about 5% of 'normal' people at this age, while focal epilepsy is very rare at the onset of a stroke.

Papilloedema

Many of the lesions which might be confused with an acute stroke cause raised intracranial pressure. Whilst the intracranial pressure may be somewhat raised after a vascular lesion, it is never sustained for long enough to produce papilloedema at the time of a patient's presentation.

The level of consciousness

Raised intracranial pressure from a mass lesion usually depresses consciousness out of proportion to any associated focal deficit. Furthermore, the conscious level tends to fluctuate. Drowsiness *may* follow a large vascular lesion but there is an appropriately substantial focal deficit as well. A large subarachnoid haemorrhage can cause drowsiness with mild or no focal signs but there is very likely to be neck-stiffness and other obvious clinical features. Another exception to the general rule is if there is direct damage to the diencephalic arousal mechanisms from occlusion of the perforating vessels from the top of the basilar artery, or from thalamic haemorrhage. Both of these types of stroke are very uncommon. Finally, haemorrhages or ischaemic lesions in the posterior fossa may cause obstructive hydrocephalus and depress the conscious level, but these patients usually show the expected cerebellar or brainstem signs. Therefore patients who present with a mild hemiparesis (or other focal deficit) and marked drowsiness may not have a stroke:

A 60-year-old man with a past history of myocardial infarction was seen by his GP after a 'blackout'. The description was vague, since his wife was out at the time and he was unable to describe the event further. There were no physical signs but he was hypertensive. An ECG was normal. Three days later the patient's wife rang to say that he had a severe frontal headache. Again there were no abnormal signs and an urgent appointment with a neurologist was arranged by the GP. Over the next 3 days the patient's wife noticed that he periodically became inexplicably drowsy and was clumsy in the use of his right limbs. Then, 6 days after the original consultation, the man was taken to hospital as an emergency after becoming unrousable at home. On arrival his conscious level had improved such that he was drowsy with a mild right hemiparesis, equivocal neck stiffness and no papilloedema.

Noting his previous history of hypertension, the hospital phys-
icians diagnosed a spontaneous intracerebral haematoma. A CT
scan, performed after his conscious level had again declined,
showed a substantial left subdural haematoma with shift of the
intracranial contents to the right (Figure 4.2).

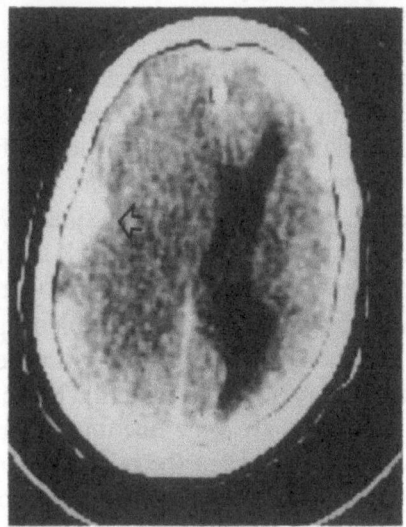

Figure 4.2   CT scan showing a left subdural haematoma (white on
the image and arrowed) and considerable shift of the intracranial
contents to the right

In this case the fluctuating conscious level was far in excess of
the degree of his hemiparesis. It is worth noting that about
50% of patients with chronic subdural haematomas have no
past history of head injury. Just because patients are hypertensive or have other risk factors for stroke does not protect
them from other brain lesions.

Combinations of suspicious features

Concurrence of one or more of the suspicious features outlined
below is a definite indication that the patient with an apparent
'stroke' should be referred for further investigation to exclude
a mass lesion:

unclear history of onset,
focal deficit progresses over more than 24 hours,
stuttering deficit,
focal or generalized seizures at onset,
depression of conscious level out of proportion to any focal
  deficit,
papilloedema,
no risk factors for stroke,
patient unusually young (age < 50).

Such combinations occur in 10% of patients with stroke, but
in up to 60% of patients with non-vascular lesions masquerading as strokes. However, vascular lesions are much
more common than the others. Therefore many of the patients
quite correctly referred for investigation will turn out to have
a vascular lesion after all. There is no way in which clinical
assessment can completely exclude a mass lesion. Rather,
clinical diagnosis should be looked on as a means of screening
the large number of patients with apparent 'stroke' to detect
the minority who have something else. Of course, if missed in
the first assessment, mass lesions will reveal themselves in the
course of time through their natural history, and usually a
slight delay is of no great consequence. The deficit associated
with mass lesions will continue to progress in the following
weeks rather than showing the tendency to improve which
characterizes most strokes. Many other non-vascular lesions
also tend to improve, including demyelination, Todd's paresis
and the focal deficits sometimes produced by hypoglycaemia.

What type of vascular lesion is present?

Vascular lesions of the brain can be divided into two pathological types: intracranial haemorrhage (subarachnoid,
primary intracerebral or both) and cerebral infarction (thrombotic or embolic). This distinction is not absolute since infarcts
may become haemorrhagic. In patients with acute stroke clinical methods are, at best, only moderately accurate in dis-

tinguishing those with intracerebral haemorrhage from the much more numerous patients with ischaemic stroke. When the consequences of mistaking an intracerebral haemorrhage for cerebral infarction are serious, such as when anticoagulation or possibly even aspirin is proposed, bedside diagnosis cannot replace the need for a CT scan. The statistical differences in the distribution of the clinical features between groups of patients with the two different types of stroke have encouraged the teaching that they can be distinguished at the bedside. In recent years several scoring systems, such as the 'Allen Score', have been devised in an attempt to use these clinical differences in a formal way. These attempts have been only partially successful. Statistical methods can only provide answers which are more or less probable rather than black and white; something which is often not good enough for the individual patient.

Subarachnoid haemorrhage

The clinical recognition of most patients with SAH is straightforward since they usually present with a distinct clinical picture. Without warning the patient develops a sudden headache, may pass out transiently, and is found to have neck stiffness (although the latter sign may take some hours to appear). Sometimes the headache is not all that severe, but it is always *sudden*. The pain may be felt in the neck rather than in the head. Vomiting occurs quite commonly. Unless there is also bleeding into the brain, there will be no focal deficit in the early stages but spasm of one or more of the main cerebral arteries may produce a focal deficit some days later. The bleeding from an intracranial aneurysm may disrupt the diencephalic structures subserving consciousness, causing persistent coma. Disruption of the hypothalamus may cause cardiovascular complications such as pulmonary oedema and subendocardial ischaemia.

Primary intracerebral haemorrhage

Only a minority of patients (about 10%) with stroke have a primary intracerebral haemorrhage and an even smaller proportion have a SAH. The clinical features of patients with intracerebral haemorrhage are often indistinguishable from those of the more numerous patients with cerebral infarction:

> A 71-year-old woman with a past history of hypertension was on a bus returning from buying a dress. She kept on dropping the dress from her left hand. On reaching home she fell to the floor without losing consciousness or vomiting. By the time she was admitted to the accident department she had developed a left hemiparesis but complained of no headache and had no neck stiffness. The stroke had evolved over a period of 1 hour from the time she first noticed the dress dropping from her hand. On admission to hospital her blood pressure was 160/100 but this fell without treatment to 140/90 after 24 hours. She remained alert throughout, and gave a clear history. She had a conjugate gaze palsy to the left and a moderately severe left hemiparesis with parietal dysfunction. There was no history of ischaemic heart disease, peripheral vascular disease or diabetes. A CT scan performed thirteen days after the onset of the stroke (Figure 4.3) showed a substantial intracerebral haematoma in the right basal ganglia.

Many of the clinical features which might help distinguish intracerebral haemorrhage from cerebral infarction are in the clinical history. Vomiting and loss of consciousness early in the course of a stroke's onset are both more frequent in intracerebral haemorrhage than infarction. Headache is only relevant if it is sudden in onset and accompanied by vomiting, loss of consciousness or neck stiffness, in which case the cause of the stroke is likely to be haemorrhagic. Hypertension was once said to be a feature indicating a haemorrhagic stroke but this is incorrect. In this context it is necessary to distinguish clearly between hypertension as a chronic disorder and the transiently high blood pressure seen after at least 80% of acute strokes. Patients with intracerebral haemorrhage tend to have

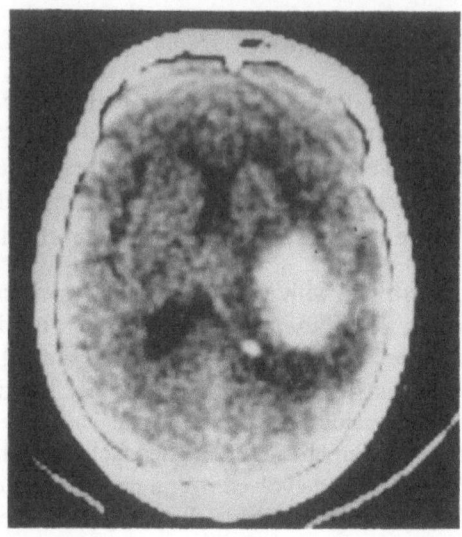

Figure 4.3   CT scan showing deep intracerebral haematoma (white on the image) in the right cerebral hemisphere

a more severe, sudden disruption of brain function than those with cerebral infarction. A haematoma in the brain acts like a sudden expanding mass lesion and the patients are more likely to show signs of general cerebral dysfunction such as depression of consciousness and bilateral extensor plantar responses. Therefore, features suggesting but certainly not proving, haemorrhage include:

loss of consciousness at onset,
sudden headache,
vomiting,
neck stiffness (meningism),
depression of conscious level within 24 hours,
bilateral extensor plantars,
sustained high blood pressure.

Unfortunately many patients with primary intracerebral haemorrhage have *none* of these features.

Cerebral infarction

The onset of the focal deficit is usually very abrupt. However, in about 20% the deficit comes on in a stuttering fashion over some minutes or hours, which is rare in patients with intracerebral haemorrhage though, as the case history above shows, it may occur. Other features which may help to distinguish an ischaemic from a primarily haemorrhagic stroke are signs and symptoms of extracranial arterial disease or cardiac disease. About 40% of patients with ischaemic cerebral lesions give a history of intermittent claudication, angina or diabetes, and about 20% have had a myocardial infarction. On the whole, signs of generalized vascular disease are less common in those with primary intracranial haemorrhage (subarachnoid or intracerebral) but, since vascular disease becomes more common with increasing age, older patients with haemorrhagic stroke may coincidentally show these features.

What is the cause of the vascular lesion?

Intracranial haemorrhage

When a patient presents with a spontaneous SAH without any focal deficit, the most likely cause is rupture of an intracranial aneurysm. These patients tend to have a more severe clinical deficit than those who bleed from an arteriovenous malformation (AVM). Patients with AVMs have often had focal or generalized seizures for years before their SAH, or have had previous minor episodes of headache and vomiting from less severe haemorrhages. Minor SAHs may be confused with migraine, but this difficulty has been overemphasised in the past. Any episode of 'migraine' accompanied by neck stiffness should be looked on with suspicion, particularly if the headache comes on suddenly. Patients with SAH may have focal signs if the bleeding has also been into the brain, which occurs especially frequently with AVMs since the vascular anomalies are often intracerebral as well as subarachnoid in location.

A primary intracerebral haemorrhage with secondary rupture into the subarachnoid space may be impossible to distinguish from one which has started in the subarachnoid space itself. Sometimes this distinction is not even possible on CT scanning. Patients with SAH should always be referred to a neurological or neurosurgical centre since secondary preventive surgery may be indicated.

Most primary intracerebral haemorrhages occur in patients with chronic hypertension and are caused by the rupture of small penetrating branches of the main cerebral arteries which perforate the base of the brain to supply the basal ganglia and internal capsule. Clinically it can be difficult to distinguish this cause from something less common such as amyloid angiopathy. Non-hypertensive causes of intracerebral haemorrhage (including bleeding dyscrasias, anticoagulants, etc. – see Chapter 2) are more likely to produce haematomas peripherally in the cerebral hemispheres rather than deep in the basal ganglia.

Cerebral infarction

Most patients have an ischaemic stroke because of atherosclerotic disease. This may cause thrombotic occlusion of the main cerebral arteries or the extracranial vessels. Alternatively emboli may arise from the main extracranial arteries in the neck and lodge in the cerebral vessels. The clinical presentation of the patient only rarely gives a clue as to which type of vascular occlusion is present. A few patients with progressive obliteration of the internal carotid artery complain of pain around the ipsilateral eye, contralateral to the focal deficit which may have evolved in a stuttering fashion. If an atheromatous plaque in the internal carotid artery has produced a deficit by embolism into the cerebral circulation there may be evidence of embolism into the retinal circulation, even if there

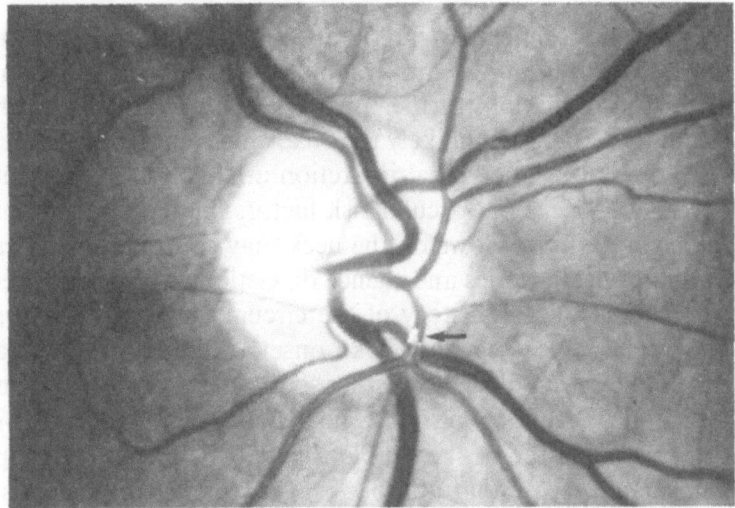

Figure 4.4 Highly refractile cholesterol embolus (arrowed) in a branch of the retinal artery in a patient with extracranial carotid artery disease

is no history of amaurosis fugax (Figure 4.4). Also, emboli may arise from the tail of a thrombus which has completely occluded an internal carotid artery.

Embolism from the heart, either from diseased valves or thrombi on the walls of the left atrium or ventricle, is a fairly common cause of cerebral infarction. However, a patient who has a potential source of embolism in the heart (see Chapter 2) may not necessarily have had a stroke for this reason. It is usually impossible to distinguish thrombotic from embolic stroke of cardiac origin by an analysis of the clinical features, despite traditional teaching that it is. The diagnosis of embolism from the heart is usually a matter of inference and circumstantial evidence. In the presence of rheumatic heart disease and atrial fibrillation, especially in a young patient, it is very likely that a stroke has been caused by embolism from the heart. However, in the case of an elderly patient with non-rheumatic atrial fibrillation it is just as likely that a stroke has been caused by atheromatous disease of the cerebral arteries.

Despite these difficulties careful attention to the examination of the heart is important. If no abnormality is found on clinical examination, further investigation of the heart with echocardiography is unlikely to reveal a relevant abnormality.

Rarer causes of cerebral infarction are likely if the patient is young and has no vascular risk factors. Sudden traction of the neck or direct blows on the neck may cause intimal tears in the cervical arteries and thence dissections which may present as a stroke. A history of the circumstances in the days and weeks preceding the stroke onset is all-important. If a carotid artery has dissected, either spontaneously or as a result of trauma, there may also be a history of pain in the neck or face preceding the stroke. In older patients a history of scalp pain may indicate that a stroke is due to giant cell arteritis. Much less commonly a younger patient may present with a stroke due to rarer types of arteritis, in which case absent pulses, infarctions in the limbs or general malaise may provide the clinical clue.

What is the extent of the damage?

In order to plan management after a stroke it is very useful to know the extent of the brain damage. The main value of this is to guide prognosis, which is of personal importance to the patient and his family, and it also influences decisions concerning referral to hospital and planning rehabilitation. Sophisticated neurological examination is not required. The types of neurological deficit found after a stroke can be summarized under five headings:

   unilateral weakness;
   unilateral sensory loss (pinprick, light touch);
   hemianopia,
   higher cerebral dysfunction;
   brainstem syndromes.

Different permutations of these main varieties of deficit describe the main presenting syndromes of stroke and allow an accurate prediction of the size of the lesion because there is a direct relationship between the syndrome and the volume of brain damage observed on CT scanning. In addition, there are some other clinical features related to the size of the lesion which can be used to increase further the accuracy of the estimation of its extent.

Uncomplicated hemiplegia (pure motor stroke)

Patients who are fully conscious and have no deficit other than weakness affecting at least two of the main areas (face, upper and lower limb) have small lesions either in the contralateral internal capsule or pons. If there is also unilateral pinprick and light touch loss (sensorimotor stroke) the lesions are slightly larger and include the thalamus. Mild dysarthria is often present, especially at the onset of the stroke but there is no cognitive deficit such as aphasia.

Pure sensory stroke

When the deficit is restricted to unilateral spinothalamic sensory loss (light touch and pinprick), the lesion is always very small and situated in the contralateral thalamus. The only functional significance of this form of stroke is that it may be complicated by a distressing syndrome of painful dysaesthesias ('thalamic pain') developing weeks or months later.

Pure hemianopia

The lesion is usually in the visual cortex if only a homonymous hemianopia is present. Deeper lesions which interrupt the optic radiations always produce additional features of parietal lobe dysfunction, in particular visuospatial neglect (see below).

Higher cerebral dysfunction

The complexity of testing for disorders of higher cerebral function is much overplayed. Quite simple screening tests take a few minutes and detect most of what is relevant.

Language. Dysphasia is detected by listening to the patient speak and asking him to name half a dozen common objects. Articulatory problems (dysarthria) should be distinguished from difficulties of language (dysphasia). Comprehension is tested by asking the patient to indicate the objects when they are described to him by the examiner. The patient may not be able to read (dyslexia) or write (dysgraphia) because of his language problem.

Inattention. Presenting simultaneous visual or tactile stimuli to both sides of the patient will detect inattention due to contralateral occipital or parietal lesions. It can also be tested by asking the patient to cross off lines drawn on a page of paper. Patients neglecting one half of their visual space will leave out the lines on that side (Figure 4.5).

Proprioception. Loss of joint position sense is usually indicative of a parietal lesion.

Isolated higher cerebral dysfunction is caused by a peripheral lesion in the posterior parietal lobe on either side (the dominant hemisphere damage being recognized by the presence of language disorder). The lesions are usually the result of occlusion of a distal branch of the middle cerebral artery, or a superfical intracerebral haemorrhage.

Higher cerebral function and hemiplegia

From the above discussion it can be seen that patients who have both hemiplegia *and* higher cerebral dysfunction must have deeper and usually larger lesions than if only one of these deficits is present.

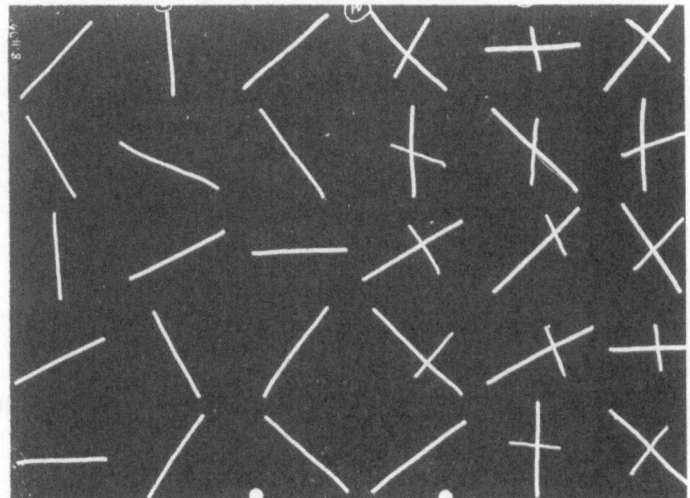

Figure 4.5 Left hemispatial neglect. The patient has been asked to cross off all the lines but has missed out those on the left (he had a large right hemisphere intracerebral haematoma)

Higher cerebral dysfunction and hemianopia

If higher cerebral dysfunction is accompanied by a homonymous hemianopia the lesion has usually involved the optic radiation under the parietal cortex.

Higher cerebral dysfunction, hemiplegia and hemianopia

This is the most severe syndrome possible, and indicates extensive cerebral hemisphere damage. The anatomical implications are of a moderate-sized deep lesion, undercutting the cortex and directly damaging the internal capsule and optic radiation. Alternatively, there may be a much larger lesion directly damaging the cortex and underlying tracts (usually a complete middle cerebral artery occlusion or large intracerebral haemorrhage).

Brainstem syndromes

Lesions in the brainstem are usually easy to recognize from the characteristic clinical features:

vertigo
diplopia
nystagmus
ataxia
persistent dysarthria
dysconjugate eye movements
(with or without unilateral or bilateral motor and sensory deficits).

The traditional practice of attempting to detect which brainstem artery is involved is a waste of time, since there are only a few specific syndromes whose recognition has any clinical relevance. These are the locked-in syndrome and cerebellar strokes.

The locked-in syndrome

This rare syndrome occurs with bilateral lesions of the brainstem, either from occlusion of the perforating branches of the basilar artery or from a pontine haemorrhage. Such lesions interrupt the motor tracts to all four limbs and, to a variable extent, the cranial nerves. However, consciousness is preserved. The patient is awake but unable to move or communicate except by signalling with vertical eye movements or blinks. It is quite easy for this state to be misinterpreted as coma, but the patient can hear and see and should be managed accordingly. If recovery occurs, which is unusual, the improvement will be noticeable in a few hours. Some patients have remained locked-in for months before eventually dying.

Cerebellar lesions with hydrocephalus

Patients with a cerebellar haemorrhage or infarct may develop hydrocephalus from pressure on the aqueduct or fourth ventricle and then obstruction of cerebrospinal fluid flow. They present with sudden imbalance and vertigo, often with vomiting and headache, and may have disorders of conjugate eye movements. However, the most important feature is deterioration in consciousness level. It is important to recognize this situation since a simple shunting procedure or evacuation of a cerebellar haematoma may save the patient's life and produce a surprisingly good functional outcome.

THE INVESTIGATION OF A PATIENT WITH ACUTE STROKE

The need for investigations depends on how accurate a diagnosis is required to ensure the best management of the patient. The routine screening investigations have already been described in Chapter 3, and the decision whether these, along with clinical assessment, are sufficient depends on what active therapeutic or preventive strategies are necessary. For some treatments, such as anticoagulation for the secondary prevention of emboli of cardiac origin, accurate diagnosis of the type of stroke is essential. After intracranial haemorrhage, determination of the cause of stroke may allow worthwhile preventive surgery to go ahead, such as clipping an intracranial aneurysm. On the other hand, in most circumstances acute treatment and preventive strategies are the same whatever the type of stroke, or are of low risk if applied to the wrong type. The treatment of stroke is discussed in Chapters 6 and 11, and a knowledge of possible and necessary treatments is an essential part of the decision whether to investigate a patient further. In this section the role of some of the available investigations will be discussed in relation to the questions they can answer.

Computerized X-ray tomography (CT scanning)

A CT scan provides a map of the structure of the brain in terms of the X-ray densities of brain tissue. Its main role is to answer the questions 'is it a mass lesion rather than a stroke?' and 'is the stroke a haemorrhage or an infarct?'. However, the proper use of the scanner to answer these questions depends on understanding the changes which occur in vascular lesions over time. At certain times after even a substantial ischaemic stroke the scan may reveal no abnormality at all. At other times the appearance of some tumours can be confused with those of an ischaemic lesion at certain stages in its evolution. Furthermore, in many stroke patients the scan is normal because the lesion is too small to be resolved (e.g. an infarct less than about 1 cm in diameter, a thin film of subarachnoid blood, brainstem strokes).

Immediately after a patient has an intracerebral haemorrhage it will be seen as an area of high density (white on the scan image) (Figure 4.3). A large haematoma distorts the surrounding brain. Abnormal collections of blood after a SAH may also show immediately after the bleed but the blood is in the basal cisterns and cortical sulci rather than within the substance of the brain (Chapter 2, Figure 2.7). The CT scan in the weeks after an intracerebral haemorrhage reflects the pathological changes. The initial high density of the blood clot fades as the haemoglobin is broken down. After 3 or 4 weeks only a small black fluid-filled hole is seen, which is similar to that resulting from a cerebral infarct. At this stage it is impossible to answer the question 'was it an infarct or haemorrhage?' on the basis of a CT scan.

Immediately after cerebral infarction the CT scan is quite likely to be entirely normal. What the scan will first detect is the gradual accumulation of water which reduces the density of the infarct and makes it progressively darker on the CT scan image (Figure 4.6). Many infarcts do not show up for 24 hours and even then the edges of the grey-black oedematous area are blurred. Some days later, as the infarcted brain swells,

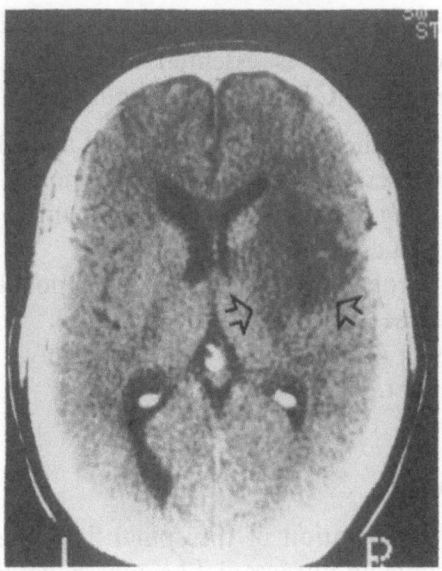

Figure 4.6 CT scan 1 week after a stroke causing a left hemiparesis and considerable left sensory neglect. Low-density area of infarction (arrowed) is clearly seen in the right cerebral hemisphere

the abnormal area on the CT scan image becomes larger and distorts the ventricular system to one side. At this point an infarct may be confused with a tumour. In the second week this oedema resolves and the mass effect disappears. By this time the infarcted area has been invaded by phagocytes which increase the X-ray density so that it may be the same as the surrounding normal brain. The CT scan, without the prior intravenous injection of contrast material, may look normal despite a marked clinical deficit. Throughout the second week and into the third the infarcted area of brain is cleared away, leaving a progressively more clearly demarcated fluid-filled hole in the brain which is shown as a clear-cut black area on the scan.

From this description it should be clear that the CT scanner can only be used to answer the questions discussed above if it is performed fairly early in the course of events. Furthermore, as with most investigative techniques, an accurate knowledge of the clinical history is essential in making an accurate interpretation of the CT images. The indications are:

1. uncertain whether the patient has had a stroke or in fact has a non-vascular brain lesion (e.g. tumour);
2. patient taking, or may need to take, anticoagulants (or possibly even aspirin);
3. cerebellar stroke (because neurosurgical possibilities);
4. SAH (because neurosurgical possibilities);
5. possibility of a later carotid endarterectomy;
6. young patient.

Lumbar puncture

In the past, examination of the spinal fluid was considered useful to exclude an intracranial haemorrhage. Bleeding into the subarachnoid space around the brain will certainly appear in the lumbar spinal fluid, as will the xanthochromic products of the degradation of its haemoglobin after some hours. A lumbar puncture is, therefore, still a useful way of confirming the clinical diagnosis of an SAH if the CT scan has not already done so. A lumbar puncture has the additional value of excluding bacterial meningitis.

After an intracerebral haemorrhage a lumbar puncture is much less accurate at detecting the haemorrhagic nature of the stroke since it is normal in the 50% or so of patients whose haemorrhage has not ruptured into the subarachnoid space. Therefore, in a patient with an acute focal stroke lumbar puncture does not usually have a role, because if it is really important to exclude an intracerebral haemorrhage a CT scan is the only way to do so reliably.

Investigating the cause of a stroke

The reason for investigating a patient after an SAH is to discover an intracranial aneurysm or arteriovenous malformation whose surgical treatment may prevent further haemorrhage. Whilst some clues as to which of these causes is present may be obtained on the CT scan, the test that answers these questions definitively is cerebral angiography. Cerebral angiography will therefore be performed if an SAH has been demonstrated by CT scanning and/or lumbar puncture, and the patient is considered to be a reasonable surgical risk.

The angiographic investigation of completed ischaemic stroke is not necessary unless some unusual pathology is suspected, such as traumatic or spontaneous arterial dissection, or unless, after a mild carotid ischaemic stroke, carotid endarterectomy is being considered (Chapter 5). After an ischaemic stroke, if a cardiac source of embolism is suspected from an ordinary clinical examination of the heart, sophisticated cardiological investigations (for example an echocardiogram) may be indicated. An ECG is always necessary to help exclude a significant arrhythmia, such as atrial fibrillation, or a recent myocardial infarct.

PRACTICAL POINTS

Mass lesions seldom mimic acute stroke and are usually identifiable by their clinical features.

The *clinical* distinction of cerebral infarction from intracerebral haemorrhage can never be completely accurate.

Simple clinical examination without complex neurological testing can accurately identify the extent of the brain damage.

CT scanning can accurately identify the type of stroke lesion present only if care is taken with its timing. It is best done within a week or so of the onset of stroke.

The distinction of cerebral infarction from primary intracerebral haemorrhage is only necessary if anticoagulants, carotid endarterectomy or (perhaps) aspirin are going to be used.

Patients with subarachnoid haemorrhage usually need further investigation in hospital.

5

NATURAL HISTORY AND TREATMENT OF TRANSIENT ISCHAEMIC ATTACKS

Most transient ischaemic attack (TIA) patients are frightened, and many are very well aware that they have just escaped having a stroke. They require sensible rather than emergency investigation, calm reassurance, and the avoidance of any sense of panic. The vast majority will be perfectly well over the next year or two even though they are at higher risk of stroke than a non-TIA patient of the same age.

The risk of stroke after TIA is *about* 5% per annum (Figure 5.1) but any stroke that does subsequently occur is not necessarily either fatal or disabling. The risk of stroke is perhaps five times that of a non-TIA population of the same age and sex. There may possibly be a rather higher risk of stroke in the first few days and weeks after a TIA. It is extremely important to think of atheromatous vascular disease in *general,* since a TIA patient is more likely to die of *cardio*vascular disease (e.g. myocardial infarction) than stroke, and the risk of myocardial infarction and/or sudden – presumed cardiac – death is much the same as the risk of stroke (Figure 5.1); cardiovascular

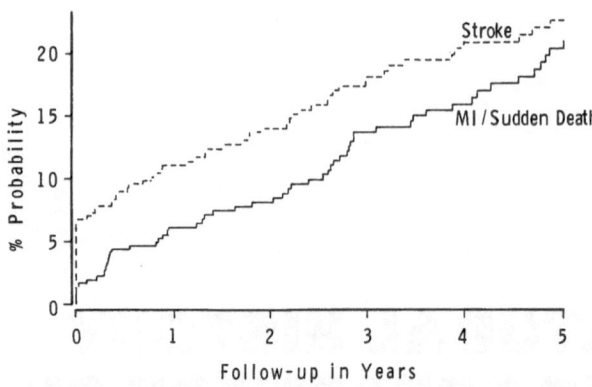

Figure 5.1 The percentage probability of stroke and myocardial infarction/sudden death over 5 years from presentation with a TIA to hospital. Most of the early high risk of stroke in this series was due not to the 'natural' history but to angiography and carotid surgery (data from 390 patients). Reproduced by permission of Dr A. Heyman and the publishers of *Neurology* (1984, **34,** 626–30)

disease is used here in a restricted sense to mean vascular disease of the heart, and not vascular disease of any organ. About 20% of TIA patients have already had symptoms of coronary artery disease, and it is hardly surprising that they are very likely to have problems such as cardiac failure, myocardial infarction, and cardiac arrhythmias. TIA are, therefore, a marker for generalized vascular disease and should not be managed merely as a risk factor for stroke.

The treatment of patients who have recovered from a focal ischaemic episode lasting minutes, hours or days is probably identical except that if it lasts days it is important to exclude an intracerebral haemorrhage by CT scanning (see Chapter 4) before starting antithrombotic – and inevitably anti-haemostatic – drugs such as warfarin and perhaps even aspirin. Another general principle is that any treatment is largely aimed at the prevention of stroke (and serious *cardio*vascular events) and not at the reduction in frequency of TIA.

TREATMENT OF EMBOLISM FROM THE HEART TO THE BRAIN

Perhaps about 10% of TIA are due to embolism from the heart to the brain rather than to the thrombotic and embolic complications of atheroma and hypertensive vascular disease (Chapter 2). This proportion is higher in the young (age < 40) where the complications of atheroma are rare; in any case TIA themselves are extremely unusual in this age group. The difficulty distinguishing a cardiac from an arterial cause of TIA has already been discussed (Chapter 3).

Patients with clear-cut mitral valve disease, either stenosis or regurgitation, with atrial fibrillation should be anticoagulated with warfarin, probably for life. The British Corrected Ratio should be maintained at about 3.0–3.5. If the TIA are very frequent (daily at least) then heparin is a reasonable treatment, at least for a few days while oral anticoagulation is being established. Patients with artificial heart valves will almost certainly already be taking warfarin, perhaps in combination with dipyridamole, and there is probably nothing further to be done unless there is a structural problem with the valve itself which only the cardiologists can sort out. If a TIA occurs within days or weeks of an acute myocardial infarct, it is probably due to embolism from left ventricular mural thrombus, and warfarin anticoagulation should be used for 3–6 months. Other less definite cardiac sources of embolism (non-rheumatic atrial fibrillation, mitral leaflet prolapse, aortic sclerosis or possibly stenosis, etc.) should probably be only treated on their *haemodynamic* merits (i.e. for cardiac failure, or arrhythmias) rather than with aspirin, or warfarin anti-coagulation.

These issues are, unfortunately, clouded by controversy, largely because there are no adequate data from clinical trials to allow rational decisions to be made. It is hardly surprising, therefore, that referral to one hospital specialist may lead a patient into the life-long rigours of warfarin treatment, while referral to another specialist leads to no more than reassurance and perhaps a little digoxin. This situation is unsatisfactory for the general practitioner and his patient, but unless we do something about it nothing will change.

ANTITHROMBOTIC DRUGS FOR TIA DUE TO THE EMBOLIC AND THROMBOTIC COMPLICATIONS OF ATHEROMA AND HYPERTENSIVE VASCULAR DISEASE

Anticoagulants

Anticoagulants were fashionable in the 1950s and 1960s for the long-term treatment of TIA despite the fact that there was, and still is, no good evidence that they influence the outcome. Anticoagulation is certainly expensive, time-consuming, and risky; TIA patients are usually elderly and often hypertensive – both factors which increase the risk of intracranial haemorrhage. Moreover, the fact that they are elderly and likely to be taking several other drugs makes the potential for drug interactions and confusion a considerable hazard. These problems *might* be worth accepting if we knew that the treatment was effective, but the evidence was so badly collected that we do not know this, and probably never will since enthusiasm for anticoagulation has waned over the last 20 years. Anticoagulation should *not*, therefore, be used for TIA patients except in the occasional case of embolism from the heart (see p. 83) and perhaps for very frequent attacks (p. 83). Naturally the normal contraindications to anticoagulant use have to be observed (peptic ulceration, severe hypertension, coagulation defects, liver disease, old age etc).

Aspirin

Aspirin causes a haemostatic defect and there is good evidence that it has a clinical effect as an antithrombotic drug. However, it is not without its problems. There is now no doubt that the higher the dose of aspirin the higher the risk of irritating gastrointestinal side-effects (indigestion, heartburn, nausea, constipation) and perhaps also the higher the risk of gas-trointestinal haemorrhage. It is also highly likely that giving aspirin inadvertently to a patient with an intracerebral haemorrhage will make matters worse, and it may even be that any cerebral infarct which occurs in someone taking aspirin becomes haemorrhagic and presumably therefore more serious.

A 70-year-old right-handed writer suddenly became dysphasic. Within a few hours his speech seemed to be normal. His general practitioner started aspirin on the assumption that he had had a TIA. Three weeks later he was seen by a neurologist. At this stage he admitted that there *was* a mild residual disability with calculations, and also spelling. Moreover, his writing was not quite so fluent as usual. A CT scan showed a small resolving haemorrhage in the left temporal lobe. Whether that haemorrhage was the cause of his stroke (*not* TIA), or was caused by the aspirin we shall never know, but presumably continuing the drug would have been unwise.

Aspirin is not, therefore, devoid of risk, and should only be given if the risk without aspirin is definitely higher from the point of view of *disabling* stroke, and myocardial infarction. On balance, it probably is indicated in *definite* TIA patients and those recovering from a mild *ischaemic* stroke and should probably be given for life. The dose is something of a guess, but 300 mg daily is reasonable. If this causes indigestion then it is worth trying the more expensive enteric-coated preparations, or reducing the dose to perhaps 75 mg daily.

There are a number of patients who cannot tolerate aspirin because of indigestion, and for them it is worth trying an enteric-coated preparation or a lower dose from the beginning. If even this causes indigestion then the aspirin should be stopped. If the patient has had any peptic ulceration within the previous 5 years or so then it is likely that aspirin will cause indigestion or even gastrointestinal bleeding. If aspirin cannot be taken then there is no point in trying dipyridamole, and one has to concentrate on the control of vascular risk factors, and perhaps vascular surgery.

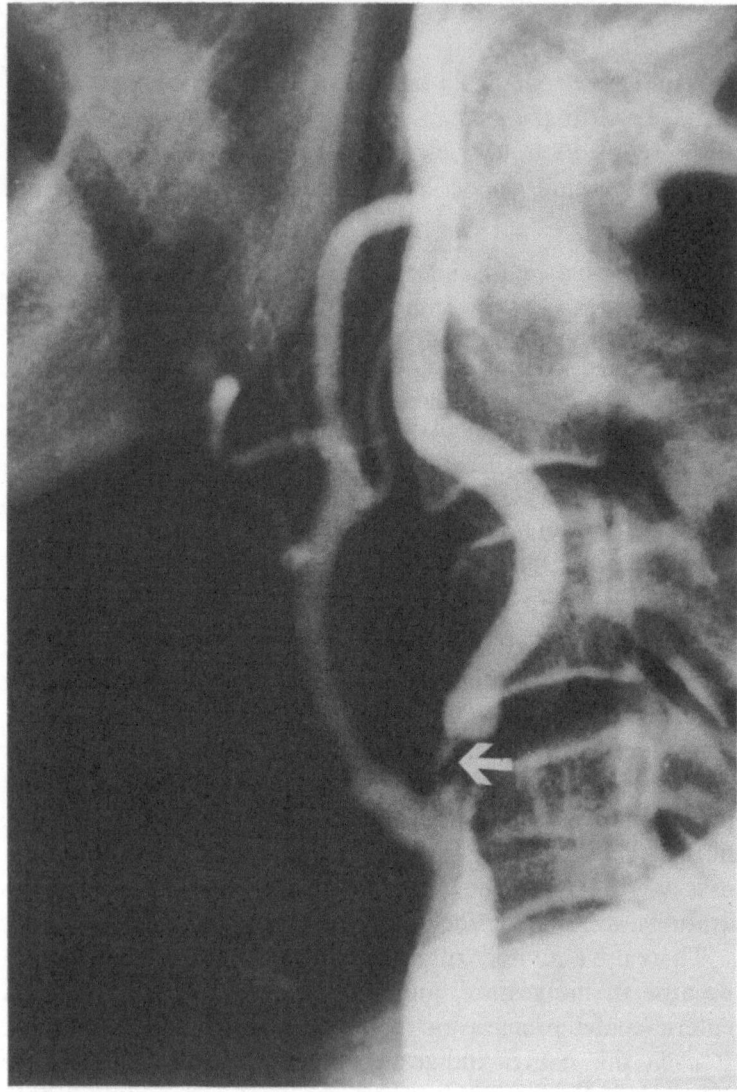

Figure 5.2 Lateral view of a carotid angiogram to show stenosis
(arrow) of the origin of the internal carotid artery

Dipyridamole (Persantin)

This is widely prescribed, usually along with aspirin, as an antithrombotic drug despite the fact that the manufacturers do not promote it for stroke prevention after TIA. There is absolutely no evidence that it is useful in TIA patients, and it should not be prescribed. It is expensive and causes some side-effects, e.g. headache.

VASCULAR SURGERY

There is some logic in the removal or bypass of stenotic, ulcerating, and occluding lesions of arteries supplying the brain and eye. A source of embolism is removed and in some cases blood flow increased. This argument applies mainly to patients who have recovered from a carotid ischaemic event (lasting minutes, hours or days) and who have stenosis (Figure 5.2) or occlusion (Figure 5.3) of the appropriate internal carotid artery (ICA) in the neck. About 40% of carotid TIA patients have stenosing lesions and about 10% have occlusions. The removal of proximal ICA stenosis is called carotid endarterectomy, while the bypass of ICA occlusion (by anastomosing a branch of the *external* carotid artery – usually the superficial temporal – through a burr hole to a distal branch of the middle cerebral artery) is called extra-cranial to intracranial (EC–IC) bypass.

Carotid endarterectomy

This operation has been performed in millions of patients over the last 30 years but there is still no evidence that it improves the patients' prognosis. Even if it does reduce the risk of stroke (by removing a source of embolism to the brain) it is unclear whether this justifies the risk of the procedure itself. The risk of angiography (which is only required as a prelude to surgery)

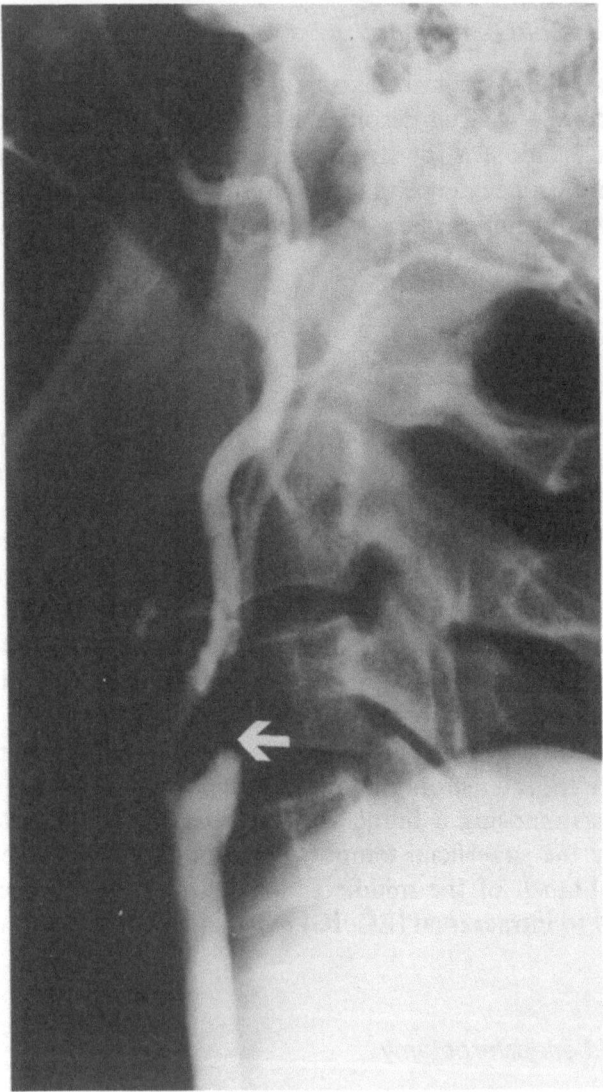

Figure 5.3   Lateral view of a carotid angiogram to show complete occlusion (arrow) of the origin of the internal carotid artery

added to the risk of the operation and anaesthetic is somewhere between 5% and 10% for stroke and/or death. The operation should only be done by an experienced surgical and anaesthetic team, and even then only if a careful audit is kept of the surgical morbidity and mortality. The evidence does not really support its use, except in the context of well-run clinical trials to find out if the operation really has any value or not.

EC–IC bypass

This procedure has been better evaluated than carotid endarterectomy, even though it is a more recently developed technique. Despite its technological elegance it does not seem to have any role in the prevention of stroke.

There are various surgical procedures for patients with vertebrobasilar ischaemia, and for those with disease of the major arteries arising from the arch of the aorta. These are all experimental with one exception: the symptoms of subclavian steal, if frequent enough to be a nuisance, can be stopped by an axillary-to-axillary artery anastomosis, or subclavian angioplasty.

THE PATIENT WITH VERY FREQUENT TIA

Some patients have TIA which are so frequent and frightening that they are prepared to take a risk from treatment to have them stopped. However, this is an unusual situation since so few patients experience more than isolated or occasional attacks. The patient with several attacks a day is distinctly unusual. In this situation 300 mg of aspirin a day should be given, and if the attacks do not stop within 48 hours the patient should be anticoagulated with heparin followed by warfarin. If the attacks stop then the warfarin can be slowly tailed off after about 3 months and replaced by long-term aspirin. If the attacks do not stop, and are in the carotid distribution, then there is some merit in at least considering carotid angiography with a view to carotid endarterectomy. On the other hand the diagnosis may be wrong, or the antithrombotic drugs ineffective anyway and should be stopped. These guidelines are very empirical because they are based on anecdotal evidence and unreliable data (in other words clinical impression).

VASCULAR RISK FACTORS

Any TIA patient must be reviewed for vascular risk factors which should be controlled on their merits in the same way as for patients without a TIA (see Chapter 10). Indeed, it may be easier to motivate a frightened TIA patient to stop smoking and comply with blood pressure reduction than an asymptomatic individual. In any event blood pressure reduction should be gradual, with particular care in patients known to have severe arterial occlusive disease in their neck. A further point is that any potential side-effects of drugs should not be ignored and misinterpreted as symptoms of the anxiety and stress of having had a TIA.

REFERRAL TO HOSPITAL

Referral to a hospital specialist is necessary if the general practitioner is uncertain about the diagnosis of TIA, uncertain of the cause of the TIA, needs an investigation which he cannot organize for himself, does not know what treatment to give, or is not in a position to manage a particular treatment. Also, the general practitioner may feel that it is easier for him to manage·the patient in the long term if he has the initial backing of a specialist. The speed of referral depends on the individual patient's problem, but a wait for more than a month for a specialist to make the diagnosis or initiate treatment is not really acceptable. Who to refer to depends on the local situation, and the general practitioner needs to know who is interested in TIA (not necessarily the visiting neurologist), and who has access to any complicated diagnostic procedures that may be required (e.g. CT scanning, angiography). Referral directly to a surgeon is unwise unless the general practitioner is extremely sure of his ground and what he is doing. One hopes that the local physician has a good enough relationship with the best available surgeon to pass on appropriate patients. For most TIA patients the general practitioner can handle the treatment *provided* he is confident with the diagnosis, and *provided* he has done a few straightforward investigations (Chapter 3).

PRACTICAL POINTS

The risk of serious *cardio*vascular events is as high as, or higher than, the risk of stroke.

Vascular risk factors should be controlled as appropriate (Chapter 10).

Other vascular problems must be dealt with on their merits, e.g. claudication, angina, cardiac failure, atrial fibrillation, aortic aneurysm, etc.

Anticoagulation with warfarin (occasionally preceded by heparin) is reasonable in patients with mitral valve disease and atrial fibrillation, recent myocardial infarction, and artificial heart valves.

Aspirin 300 mg daily is reasonable in patients who have TIA as a result of atherothromboembolism.

Dipyridamole should not be used except in the case of prosthetic heart valves.

Vascular surgery is controversial, and the decision should really be left to the local neurologist.

Very frequent TIA occurring more than once a day should be treated with aspirin, or if that fails with anticoagulation. If that fails then the treatment should be stopped, carotid endarterectomy considered perhaps, and the diagnosis reconsidered as well.

6

THE NATURAL HISTORY AND TREATMENT OF STROKE

Most large studies of the natural history of stroke are based on patients admitted to hospital and may, therefore, be of limited value to the general practitioner. The aim of this chapter is to describe the natural history of all stroke in the community and not just in hospital, highlight certain features which influence management, discuss the benefits or otherwise of various potential treatments, and then discuss the long-term prognosis. The natural history is usually described in two parts – 'early' – i.e. within 30 days of the stroke, and 'late'. Although this division is arbitrary, it corresponds to a flattening of the case fatality curve (Figure 6.1).

EARLY PHASE

In about 60% of patients the focal neurological deficit is maximal either on waking or within an hour of the onset of symptoms. Less than 10% progress for more than 24 hours, so-called 'stroke-in-evolution' or 'progressing stroke'. Impair-

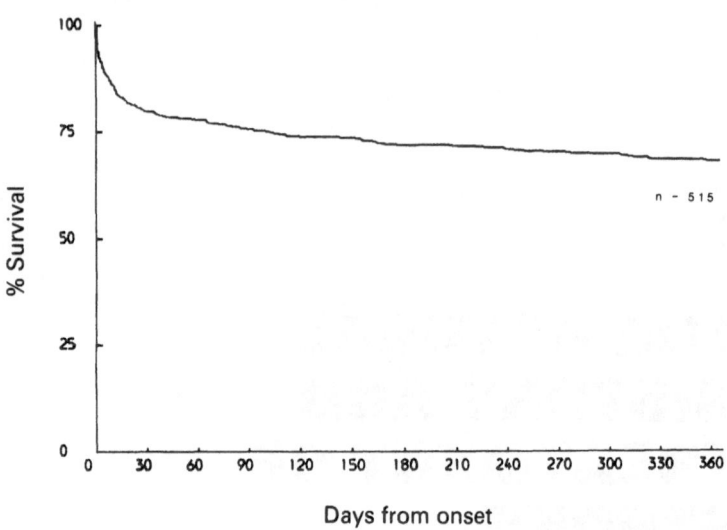

Figure 6.1   One-year survival curve after first-ever stroke based on 515 patients in the Oxfordshire Community Stroke Project, 1981–4

ment of conscious level within a few hours of the onset is unusual, and suggests that either the stroke is haemorrhagic, or that the brainstem or cerebellum is involved, or that the diagnosis is not stroke.

Early case fatality

How many deaths?

Community-based studies suggest that about 20% of patients having a first stroke will die within 30 days of the onset. If patients with recurrent strokes are included this figure rises to between 25% and 30%. This contrasts with the rates reported in hospital-based studies, which are as high as 50% because more severe strokes tend to be admitted to hospital. The 30–day case fatality rate differs widely between stroke types, intracranial haemorrhage clearly being more lethal than cerebral infarction (Figure 6.2).

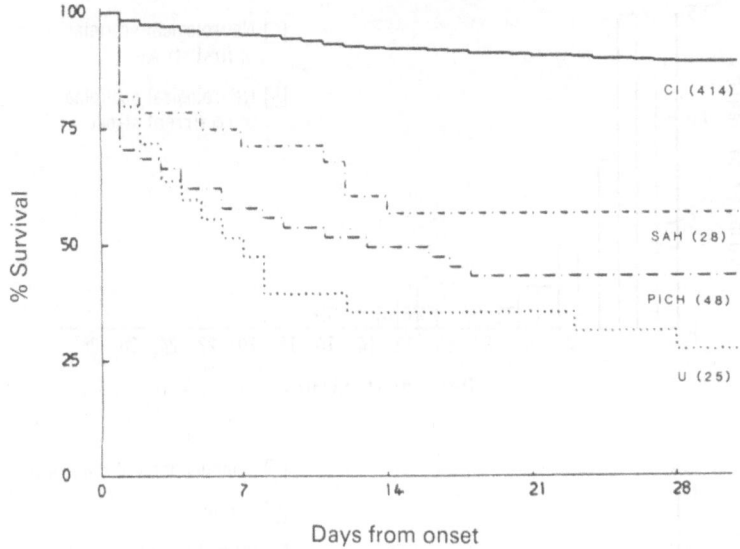

Figure 6.2 Thirty-day survival curve by stroke type based on 515 patients with first-ever stroke in the Oxfordshire Community Stroke Project (1981–4). CI = cerebral infarction; SAH = subarachnoid haemorrhage; PICH = primary intracerebral haemorrhage; and U = uncertain pathology

Early deaths – when and why?

Analysis of the timing and cause of death is important if rational decisions are to be made about treatment. Causes of death can be considered in four groups: (1) direct neurological sequelae of the stroke, e.g. transtentorial herniation, or disruption of brainstem respiratory and cardiovascular centres; (2) complications of immobility, e.g. pneumonia, pulmonary embolism, sepsis; (3) cardiac disease and (4) other disorders not directly related to the stroke, such as renal failure. Fifty per cent of the early deaths occur within the first week post-stroke and the vast majority of these are due to 'neurological' factors. The timing and cause of deaths within the first 30 days post-stroke are shown in Figure 6.3.

Death within 24 hours of the onset of symptoms is extremely unusual. When it does occur the stroke is usually either a

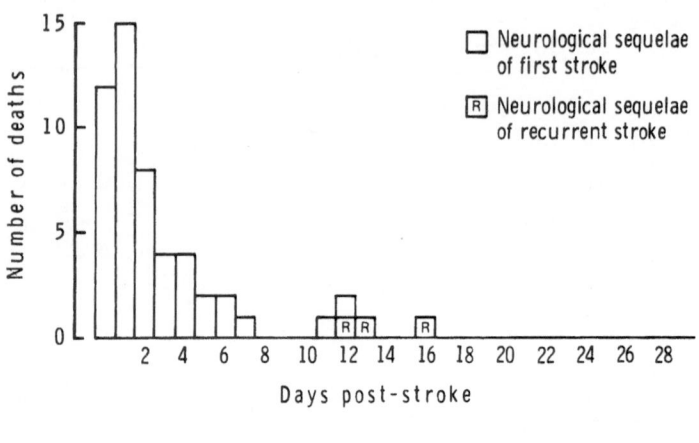

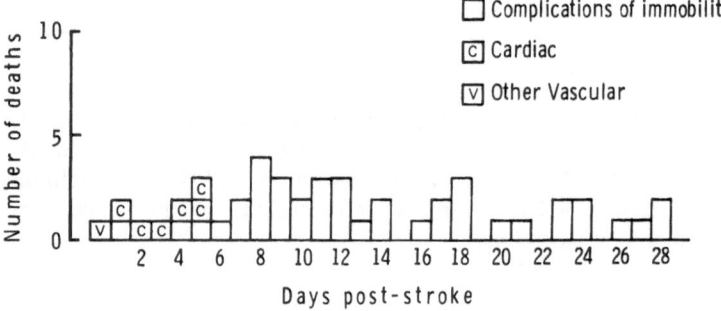

Figure 6.3 Timing and cause of early deaths in the patients dying within 30 days from 515 first-ever strokes in the Oxfordshire Community Stroke Project (1981–4). Above are the 'neurological' deaths directly due to the intracerebral haemorrhage or cerebral infarct, and below are the 'non-neurological' deaths which are usually an indirect consequence of the cerebral lesion

major subarachnoid haemorrhage, a massive supratentorial intracerebral haemorrhage, or an infratentorial haemorrhage, in particular cerebellar haemorrhage. Infarction in the brain-stem may cause death within the first 72 hours by directly compromising the respiratory and cardiovascular centres. Deaths due to transtentorial herniation from supratentorial infarcts tend to occur slightly later.

In patients surviving the first week, the most likely cause of death within the next 3 weeks is one of the complications of immobility. Deaths due to cardiac disease are probably equally distributed throughout the time period though recognition of this may be dependent on the level of monitoring employed.

Prediction of early death

The important factors associated with an increased risk of early death are shown in Figure 6.4. Impairment of conscious level is the best predictor of early death, although other features such as gaze paresis, bilateral extensor plantar responses, and pupillary abnormalities are also signs of a poor prognosis. There is an increased case fatality rate with increasing age (Figure 6.5), but this is apparent only after the first week, suggesting that elderly patients are more likely to succumb to the complications of immobility rather than that they are more susceptible to the direct neurological sequelae of the stroke itself.

ACUTE TREATMENT

If one considers the underlying mechanisms causing stroke it is easy to think of therapeutic interventions which might be expected to reduce the mortality, extent or complications of the stroke, and it is easy to find reports in the literature to support virtually any hypothesis. What is almost universally lacking are controlled trials of an adequate size which show a significant benefit as a result of *any* form of intervention. Although this smacks of therapeutic nihilism, it is usually because trials have not been performed at all, rather than that trials have been done which did not show any definite benefit. Even the few trials that have been done were far too small to have had a reasonable chance of showing substantial treatment effects, if such effects were really there to be demonstrated.

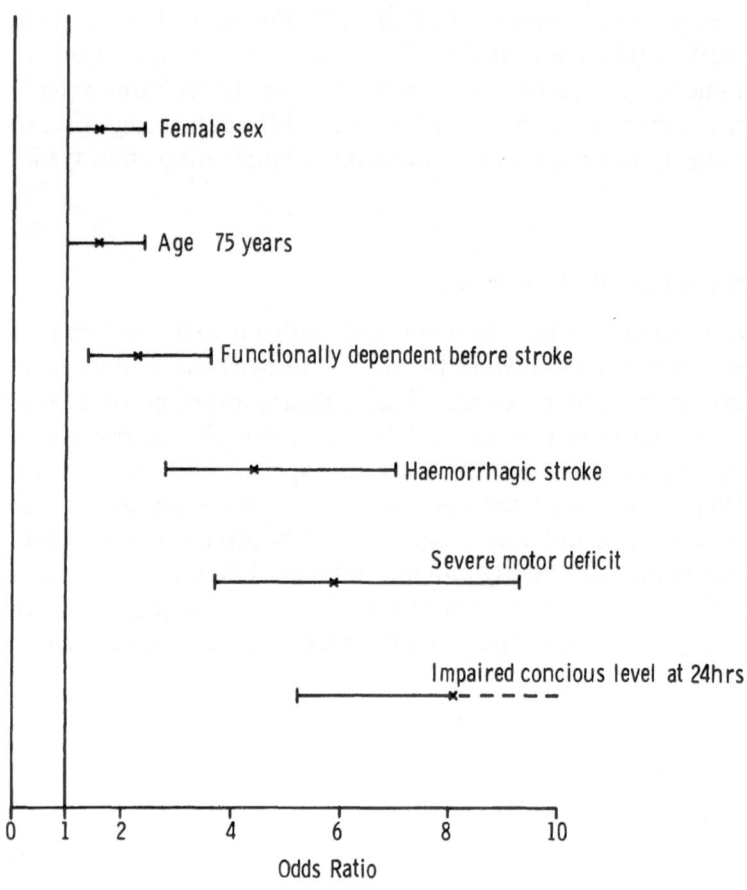

Figure 6.4 Factors associated with an increased risk of early death in the same patients as in Figures 6.2 and 6.3. The odds ratio is the odds of a patient *with* a particular factor (e.g. age > 75) dying, divided by the odds of a patient *without* a particular factor dying (e.g. age < 75). An odds ratio of one means that the factor makes no difference to early death. In the figure the crosses are the odds ratios and the horizontal bars represent the 95% confidence limits (i.e. given the sample size, the true effect is 95% likely to be somewhere along the horizontal lines)

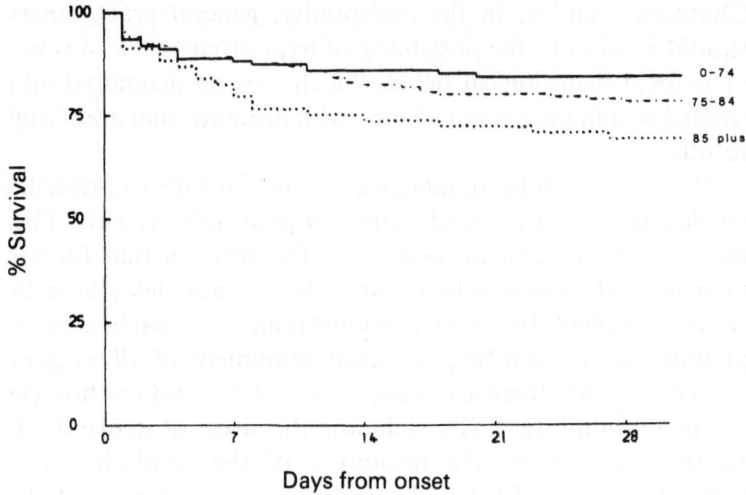

Figure 6.5 Thirty-day survival rate by age in the same patients as in Figures 6.2–6.4

Another major failing may be that insufficiently homogeneous groups of patients are considered for trials – most potential treatments are only theoretically appropriate for a particular subgroup of patients which can be difficult to identify reliably.

The following discussion will consider those treatments which are most frequently proposed, and also those which are the most promising and worth testing in future trials. They will be considered under four headings: (1) those aiming to treat a specific disease process which may have caused the stroke, (2) those that are potentially lifesaving, (3) those aiming to reduce the area of damage, and (4) those aiming to reduce the complications of immobility.

Treatment of the specific causes of stroke

The clinical features and relevant investigations to identify the very few *treatable* causes of stroke have been described in

Chapters 3 and 4. In the community, general practitioners should be alert to the possibility of hypoglycaemia as a cause of a focal neurological deficit which can be diagnosed and treated within the patient's home with dramatic and gratifying results.

There seems to be an increasing trend for GPs to prescribe corticosteroids in cases of *suspected* giant cell arteritis. This has been prompted, no doubt, by the concern that further neurological damage may occur if there is any delay in instituting treatment. However, one must remember that headache, at times severe, is a frequent accompaniment of *all* types of stroke, and that there are many causes of a raised erythrocyte sedimentation rate (ESR) including the stress of stroke itself. In the latter cases, the resolution of the headache, normalization of the ESR and the general improvement of the patient's health may occur in spite of, rather than because of, the steroids. One may then be faced with a patient on relatively high doses of steroids in whom the 'therapeutic trial' provides the only support for a diagnosis which has far-reaching implications for the patient. The value of having a tissue diagnosis cannot be overemphasized, and patients with suspected giant cell arteritis should be referred for temporal artery biopsy if at all possible, certainly within a few days of starting corticosteroids.

In cases of suspected bacterial endocarditis, antibiotics should not be given in the community as the patients require full bacteriological investigation and cardiological assessment.

Lifesaving measures

The early case fatality rate of stroke is between 20% and 30%, and only about half the deaths are due to the direct neurological sequelae of the stroke. This means that in a practice covering 10 000 people only about two patients every year will die for this reason. Neurological deaths occur due to disruption of the brainstem respiratory and cardiovascular centres and are usually preceded by progressive impairment of consciousness. They may be due to direct disruption by intrinsic brainstem lesions, transtentorial herniation and brainstem compression due to large supratentorial infarcts or haematomas, or compression of the brainstem by expanding infratentorial lesions (which usually have the added complication of acute hydrocephalus). Consequently, it is unlikely that any one form of treatment will be appropriate in all cases. When considering potential treatments aimed at saving life, the issue of what quality of life is saved must be addressed as well; survival in a hopelessly disabled state is presumably not a desirable outcome for a treatment that 'works' by saving lives.

Medical

Deaths from transtentorial herniation due to the oedema surrounding large cerebral infarcts tend to occur 2–7 days post-stroke. Anti-oedema agents, in particular mannitol, may reduce mortality but the long-term prognosis for functional recovery is poor so that the justification for such intervention is questionable. It may be thought that corticosteroids should be beneficial in stroke patients because of the dramatic effect they have on the oedema surrounding tumours. However, several studies using various doses of steroids have failed to show any beneficial effect. This may be because the oedema surrounding tumours is primarily 'vasogenic', that is arising from the breakdown of the blood–brain barrier, whilst that around strokes is 'cytotoxic' as well, and more to do with the breakdown of cell membranes.

Surgery

Patients with a rapidly declining level of consciousness within 24 hours of the onset of symptoms are likely to have had an intracerebral haemorrhage and the question of surgery arises.

The only situation in which there is reasonably convincing evidence of the efficacy of surgical treatment is with cerebellar haemorrhage when either the haematoma may be evacuated, or the accompanying acute hydrocephalus relieved with a shunt (Figure 6.6). The rapid progression of this type of stroke often means that, apart from impaired level of consciousness, there are few other obvious signs; this clinical conundrum may be summed up by the aphorism 'stroke somewhere, stroke nowhere, stroke in the cerebellum'. Any individual GP is unlikely to encounter this type of stroke more than once in a career, but should nevertheless remain acutely aware of its potentially treatable nature. A similar, although generally less acute, situation can occur with extensive cerebellar infarction. The best outcome after surgery is in patients who are still conscious at the time of operation; therefore rapid referral to a neurosurgical centre is vital.

The surgical management of supratentorial haematomas, although attractive technically, is of unproven value. Good

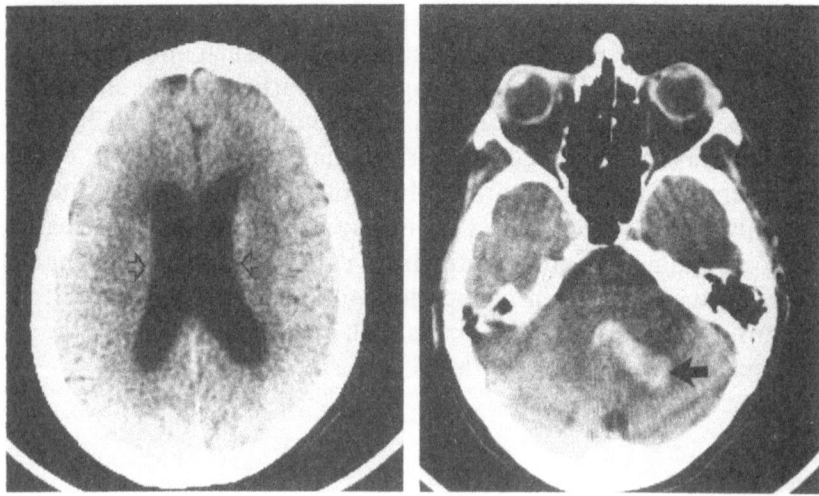

Figure 6.6   CT scan of a cerebellar haematoma (white area arrowed) on the right panel; on the left is a higher cut showing hydrocephalus with enlargement of the lateral ventricles (arrowed)

survival has been reported in patients with superficial hae-matomas who were conscious at the time of operation, but many of these would have survived anyway. There is no evidence that the extent of residual deficit is lessened by surgery. It should *possibly* be considered in patients with progressive impairment of conscious level.

Restriction of the area of damage

Cerebral infarction occurs due to either the partial or total interruption of the local blood supply. A totally ischaemic area probably remains viable only for a few minutes, but within the distribution of an occluded artery the degree of ischaemia is not uniform due to collateral circulation. Areas with relative ischaemia, though functionally impaired, may remain viable, and therefore potentially salvageable, for several days. However, in such areas, because of the reduced supply of oxygen, there may be a switch to anaerobic metabolism. The subsequent production of lactic acid may damage cell membranes and cause extension of the infarct and cerebral oedema, accompanied by loss of normal vascular auto-regulation. Positron emission tomography has shown that the normal response is to extract more oxygen from the blood and to open up collateral vessels, though the mechanisms controlling such processes are obscure. Various treatments, some more rational than others, have been suggested to 'rescue' these functionally impaired areas.

For a GP intending to manage a patient with stroke at home, there are two broad ways in which, potentially, the area of damage may be limited: either by alteration of variables such as blood pressure, blood viscosity and glucose; or by the use of specific therapeutic agents. At present it is the former group which is more promising.

Blood pressure

The control of blood pressure around the time of a stroke raises considerable theoretical problems, and the fact that chronically raised blood pressure is a risk factor for stroke should not be confused with its management in the acute phase. The loss of vascular autoregulation in and around an infarct means that the perfusion pressure has a large influence on the cerebral blood flow. Firstly, therefore lowering blood pressure, particularly suddenly, may actually lead to *reduced* perfusion. Secondly, many patients will have a degree of major extracranial artery stenosis, and flow across this stenosis may also rely on a relatively high perfusion pressure. Thirdly, patients with chronically raised blood pressure have altered autoregulation, and determining what their previously 'normal' pressure was may be extremely difficult, though the GP is often better placed to know this than a hospital doctor. Blood pressure is often very labile around the time of stroke, especially if brainstem structures are involved, and isolated recordings are an unreliable guide to the mean pre-stroke pressure level.

It is reasonable to leave patients already on antihypertensives on their medication as long as the blood pressure is near 'normal' for that individual (something which the GP is ideally placed to know). For the vast majority of patients the *initiation* of antihypertensive treatment should usually be delayed by a week or so to allow the blood pressure to stabilize.

It is clear that over-enthusiastic use of antihypertensive agents in the acute phase is likely to result in *increased* damage, and therefore should in general be avoided. The major exception is in patients with accelerated or malignant hypertension who have retinal haemorrhages, exudates, papilloedema or haematuria, in which case cautious reduction of blood pressure should be initiated, preferably in hospital and with oral rather than intravenous agents.

The effect of raising the blood pressure (as a means of increasing blood flow to the ischaemic penumbra of cerebral infarcts where there is failure of vascular autoregulation) has not been tested in detail, though a number of anecdotal reports have suggested benefit.

Hyperglycaemia

There is some evidence that hyperglycaemia increases the area of infarction and oedema because glucose, the metabolic substrate for brain metabolism, is being provided in the absence of adequate oxygen delivery. This promotes anaerobic metabolism and the production of lactic acid, which is possibly neurotoxic. No trials have shown that inducing relative hypoglycaemia is of benefit, but it would seem reasonable to try and maintain normoglycaemia. Many patients have a transient rise in blood sugar, presumably related to the stress of the stroke.

Blood viscosity

There is no evidence that routinely reducing blood viscosity, either by venesection and/or infusion of agents such as dextran, significantly reduces the area of infarction or the resulting functional disability. If a patient has polycythaemia rubra vera, then reduction of the haematocrit and viscosity to more normal values would seem sensible, though venesection should be performed with caution, especially in the elderly.

Anticoagulants

Anticoagulants are probably the group of drugs most frequently considered in patients with acute stroke. Various ways in which this treatment might work have been proposed, including the prevention of complete occlusion of a stenotic artery, prevention of further embolic events either from the heart or from thrombotic lesions in the major extracranial vessels, and prevention of the propagation of thrombus above an occlusion in an extracranial artery. As discussed in Chapter 4, although the technology exists to distinguish haemorrhagic from ischaemic strokes, there are no easy ways of detecting most of the pathological mechanisms underlying infarction, so even if anticoagulants were really beneficial in one of these subgroups of infarcts, it would not be surprising if trials which included *all* cerebral infarcts failed to show that anticoagulation was effective.

Anticoagulants have a serious complication rate, which may be as high as 4%. The risks are known to increase with age and hypertension, both of which have a high prevalence amongst patients with stroke. The problem of haemorrhagic transformation of infarcts has not been widely studied. About 5% of infarcts become haemorrhagic spontaneously, and it has been suggested that large infarcts, and those due to embolic occlusion of the major vessels, are the most likely to do so. In the latter case it is thought that disintegration of the embolus allows the full systemic blood pressure to be exerted on the relatively fragile ischaemic tissues. Of course it is precisely this type of stroke for which anticoagulation is most likely to be considered. The risk of haemorrhagic transformation in patients on anticoagulants may be about 10%, though it is not known whether this makes any difference to the outcome.

In general, the use of anticoagulants as a means of restricting cerebral damage is unproven, and is not without considerable risks. There are a number of small, poorly conducted trials that suggest benefit from anticoagulation in cases of progressing stroke. Defining such cases is difficult, but a patient showing a stepwise neurological deterioration might be considered in this category. Pathological evidence suggests that occlusion of the extracranial carotid and vertebral arteries may occur in several stages, and *if* this could be correlated with the clinical syndrome of progressing stroke then anticoagulants *may* have some benefit. The number of such patients is small, but there may be value in identifying them. If anticoagulation is being considered (for example in cases of rheumatic atrial fibrillation) then the patients must be very closely observed, and CT scanning facilities must be available (see Chapter 4).

Fibrinolytic agents

There is no evidence to support the use of fibrinolytic agents such as streptokinase or urokinase in patients with stroke. The small number of cases reported suggest that such treatment is detrimental and causes intracranial haemorrhagic complications.

Vasodilators

There have been a number of reports (often followed by intensive drug marketing) proposing that vasodilators may limit the area of damage, theoretically by allowing more flow through collateral vessels. A similar rationale lay behind the use of inhalation of 5% carbon dioxide and stellate ganglion block. The fallacy of this argument is that, with the loss of autoregulation around an infarct, most vessels are maximally dilated anyway, and these measures might divert blood flow *away* from the infarct. There is no evidence that any vasodilator is of value.

Surgical revascularization

Acute surgical procedures such as carotid endarterectomy or extracranial–intracranial bypass are sometimes suggested as a means of restoring blood flow to ischaemic areas, but they have a high perioperative mortality and are not recommended.

Prevention of complications

Between 20 and 40% of early deaths are due to complications
of immobility such as pneumonia, pulmonary embolism and
sepsis. The prevention of such complications owes more to
common-sense management, which can be done in the patient's home, than controlled trials of specific therapies.

Respiration

Any reduction in oxygenation is likely to be detrimental to the
patient; therefore prompt treatment of chest infections with
antibiotics and physiotherapy, which can often be taught to
relatives if domiciliary services are stretched, is important –
assuming that the patient is likely to survive the stroke. In
general, protection of the airway by intubation and assisted
ventilation is unlikely to benefit the patient in the long-term,
though it should be considered in patients with brainstem
strokes whose prognosis, should they survive the acute event,
may be relatively good.

Dysphagia

Transient dysphagia is common and does not necessarily mean
that the stroke has involved brainstem structures. It usually
recovers in a few days, and during this time the patient should
be managed with sufficient clear fluids to maintain reasonable
hydration (1.5–2 litres daily). It is rarely necessary to resort to
nasogastric feeding or intravenous fluids.

Bedsores and incontinence

A good standard of nursing care is required to prevent disabled
patients developing bedsores and secondary sepsis. However,

in many cases such nursing will only be required for a few days, and clear instructions to relatives about turning and positioning along with the *rapid* provision of aids such as sheepskins may allow the patient to remain at home. Urinary incontinence is often transient, and sheath urinals and incontinence pads may prevent the need for catheterization with all the attendant risks of urine infection.

Deep vein thrombosis and pulmonary embolism

Deep vein thrombosis, either clinically apparent or silent, occurs in about 50% of immobilized stroke patients leading to death from pulmonary embolism in a few cases. It has been suggested that low-dose subcutaneous heparin may reduce the incidence of such events, though an adverse effect on primary intracerebral haemorrhage or haemorrhagic infarction is possible. This treatment should not be used routinely, and certainly not before a CT scan has ruled out intracranial haemorrhage.

Summary of acute treatment – now and the future

It is clear by considering the pathophysiology of stroke that it is almost inconceivable that any one treatment will be beneficial to all patients. This point has often been overlooked in the past when trials have been conducted, and may in fact have led to the premature abandonment of treatments beneficial to one subgroup. It is likely that trials in the future will take this factor into account, but investigators must define clearly the patients to whom any treatment is applicable, preferably based on clinical findings rather than high technology and impractical investigations. The GP's role will then include the identification of these patients and either initiation of the treatment, or referral for further investigations. Currently, GPs should try and identify those few patients with arteritis and other treatable causes of stroke, cerebellar lesions, and progressing

stroke particularly since some of the last turn out to have
intracranial space-occupying lesions.

The acute management of patients who do not fall into such
categories, which at present means the vast majority, should
be based on a common-sense approach to factors such as
blood pressure, blood sugar, blood viscosity and oxygenation.
The prevention of complications requires attention to details
of the patient's environment and, although this may seem less
'medical' than the use of drugs, it is likely to be considerably
more beneficial to the patient. A strong argument can be made
that the GP who knows the patient, the family and the home
environment is ideally placed to do this, perhaps with help
from a hospital-based but community-orientated stroke team.

LONG-TERM PROGNOSIS

Recurrent stroke

In general the rate of recurrent stroke is approximately 10%
per year, and this remains relatively constant over several
years. It is frequently stated that if recurrence is going to occur
it will do so soon after the stroke. Although this may be true
amongst certain subgroups of stroke, in the acute phase it is
often difficult to decide whether a patient is having a recurrent
event or merely a stuttering onset of the initial stroke. For this
reason some authors discuss recurrence rates in relation to
those patients who have survived 1 month after their stroke,
and this is probably more relevant to the GP who may be
dealing with patients after their discharge from hospital. The
only type of stroke where the risk of recurrence is convincingly
lower than other types is subarachnoid haemorrhage. This presumably reflects the very localized pathological process causing the stroke, and the beneficial effects of surgery. One might
expect patients with cerebral infarction to have a higher recurrence rate than those with primary intracerebral haemorrhage.
There are problems interpreting the data relating to the latter
because of the relatively small numbers in all studies; however,

at the present time no convincing difference has been described. There is an increased case fatality rate amongst patients with recurrent strokes, perhaps as high as 30% in the first 30 days.

Patients who have multiple small infarcts sometimes develop a characteristic syndrome of mental impairment and a gait disturbance which has many of the qualities of extrapyramidal disease. There is often little in the way of focal limb deficit. The frequency with which this clinical picture develops is unclear.

The risk factors and prevention of recurrent stroke are discussed later.

Case fatality

The overall 1-year case fatality rate is between 30 and 40% (Figure 6.1). However, many of the patients are elderly and have coexisting disease, particularly of the heart. The effect of age on the 1-year case fatality rate is shown in Figure 6.7. Therefore any comparisons should be made with age- and sex-matched groups free from stroke. The Framingham study showed that the long-term case fatality rate of stroke patients free of cardiac disease was actually very similar to that of a matched stroke-free population.

Cause of death

With increasing time after the stroke the accuracy of the details of death dwindles. It becomes difficult to work out whether deaths are related to stroke disability or just to ageing, although it is clear that many deaths are due to cardiac disease and few are due to recurrent stroke. This has clear implications for secondary prevention and the overall management of the patient (see Chapter 11).

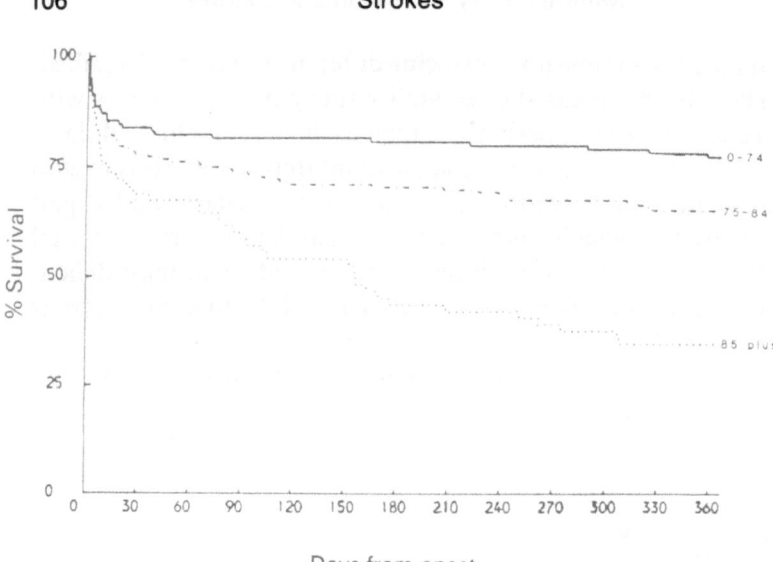

Figure 6.7 One-year survival by age in the 515 first-ever strokes in the Oxfordshire Community Stroke Project (1981–4)

Pattern of recovery

There are many problems in measuring outcome. One must make the distinction between disability and handicap – the former describes loss of function whilst the latter describes how such a loss affects the patient's life. From a practical point of view it is the assessment of handicap, rather than disability, that will be of most relevance to the GP. The crudest assessment of handicap is whether the patient is functionally independent or not. Of survivors to 1 month, between 50 and 60% are functionally independent, rising to between 60 and 70% at 6 months. This proportion then remains static. Not surprisingly, those with an extensive neurological deficit initially are most likely to remain dependent and show least recovery. This pattern of recovery does not seem to be influenced by the pathological type of stroke (Figure 6.8). The various features which predict the degree of recovery are described in Chapter 7.

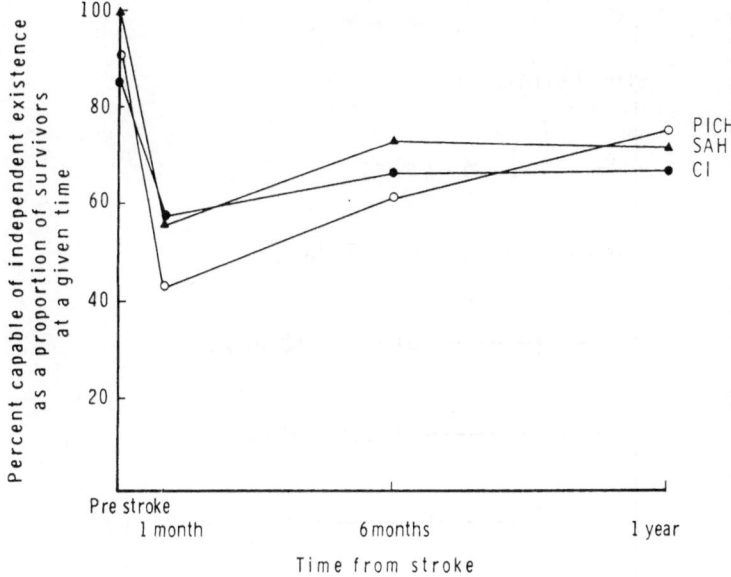

Figure 6.8   Pattern of recovery in survivors by stroke type in the 515 first-ever stroke patients in the Oxfordshire Community Stroke Project (1981–4). CI = cerebral infarction; PICH = primary intra-cerebral haemorrhage; SAH = subarachnoid haemorrhage. Note that up to 15% of patients are already dependent before the stroke. 'Independence' is rated as 0–2 on the modified Rankin scale (Appendix 2) and 'dependence' as 3–5

HOME OR HOSPITAL

In the UK between 50 and 70% of patients with acute stroke are admitted to hospital, though this figure is probably higher in urban areas. From the evidence presented in previous chapters, the number of patients requiring admission for diagnosis or specific treatment is very small. The provision of nursing or general (non-medical) care is by far the most common reason for GPs to request admission. Other factors which influence admission are shown in Figure 6.9.

The domiciliary services which are available to any individual GP vary widely; therefore the pros and cons of hospital admission can only be discussed in broad outline. It seems

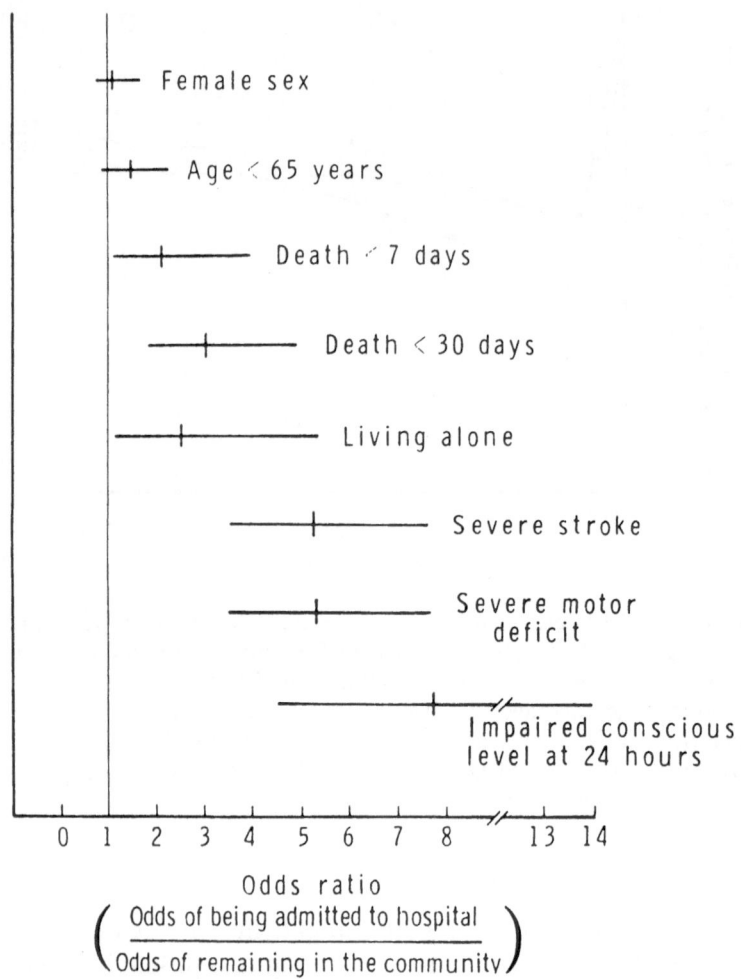

Figure 6.9 Factors influencing admission to hospital in 515 first-ever stroke patients in the Oxfordshire Community Stroke Project (1981–4). The horizontal bars are 95% confidence limits of the odds ratios (for explanation see Figure 6.4 legend). Reproduced by permission of the editor of the *British Medical Journal* (1986, **292,** 1371)

that apart from the few patients who need specific treatments most patients with stroke *could* be managed in the community. The main question is 'where will the patient get the best care, both physical and psychological, in the acute stage and during the rehabilitative phase'? There is no evidence that patients who are admitted to hospital during the acute phase recover any faster or more completely than those remaining in the community; many patients, especially the elderly, often want to stay at home with their family. One must be aware, however, that it is easy to neglect a patient at home. Nowadays, when there is pressure for increasing the proportion of patients managed at home, stroke patients may actually be a group who would benefit from such a policy, though there is no evidence that *adequate* community care is any less expensive than hospital care.

In the final analysis each patient's case has to be considered on its merits. Progress towards reducing the present dichotomy between hospital and community care is likely to benefit the patients in the long term.

PRACTICAL POINTS

Care must be taken in extrapolating from hospital-based studies which tend to report selected groups of patients with stroke who frequently have a worse prognosis compared with strokes in the community.

Impairment of consciousness within an hour of onset is rarely seen in stroke.

Overall, between 20% and 30% of patients will die within 30 days of a stroke, though intracranial haemorrhage is much more likely to be lethal than cerebral infarction. Of these, about half will die within a week due to extensive neuronal damage, whilst later deaths are more likely to be due to cardiac disease or complications of immobility.

Grave prognostic features include early impairment of consciousness, pupillary abnormalities and bilateral extensor plantar responses. The elderly are more likely to succumb to complications of immobility.

Treatable causes of stroke such as giant cell arteritis, bacterial endocarditis and embolism from rheumatic heart disease are unusual but should always be looked for, as well as the rare patient who deteriorates after a cerebellar stroke when surgery may be both lifesaving and allow a good functional outcome.

No other medical and surgical treatments of acute stroke have *yet* been shown to be of benefit. Careful control of the patient's blood pressure, biochemistry and the rapid provision of nursing support are, at present, more likely to be of benefit.

The risk of recurrent stroke is about 10% per annum. One year case fatality rate is between 30% and 40% and many of the later deaths are due to conditions unrelated to the stroke, particularly cardiac disease.

About two-thirds of survivors will be independent in activities of daily living.

Patients with stroke are most likely to be admitted to hospital in order to obtain adequate nursing care, especially if they live alone, or if the diagnosis is in doubt. The proportion of patients admitted in different places varies and will depend on many factors including the availability of domicillary services. We do not know if functional outcome is affected by hospital admission.

7

REHABILITATION

Patients with an acute stroke present their general practitioner with a succession of challenging problems: those of diagnosis (Chapter 4) and medical management (Chapter 6) have already been covered, and strategies for secondary prevention follow (Chapter 11). This chapter covers the phase from the first few days to the end of the first year; the period of recovery and rehabilitation when initial high hopes are sometimes dashed, and when patients and their families may despair.

Successful management of the disabilities caused by stroke requires close attention to detail, awareness of the natural history and chance of recovery, surprisingly little knowledge of neurology but a good knowledge of the services available locally. Unless otherwise stated, no distinction is drawn between the various types of stroke, because management is based primarily on observed disabilities rather than neuropathology or neurophysiology.

The GP, leading the primary health care team, is in the ideal position to manage acute stroke. Patients and relatives usually expect the GP to *do* something, and some GPs respond to this pressure by admitting patients to hospital. However, few patients require admission for specific reasons of diagnosis or treatment. But there are plenty of other things for the GP to *do*, even if most are 'organizational' and 'supporting', rather than giving active drug treatment. The GP can often be associ-

ated with the dramatic early stages when most survivors make
a considerable improvement. This early bonding with the
patient and family is important since many survivors will be
left with continuing problems needing attention. Further, the
GP usually knows the family best and, as stroke can have
major effects upon the whole family (Chapter 9), is in a key
position to help. This chapter provides guidance on the
rehabilitation of patients at home after acute stroke.

THE FIRST VISIT

The first decision is whether to admit the patient to hospital.
Identification of patients who need admission for diagnosis or
treatment has been discussed in Chapter 6. Where the issue is
rehabilitation, there is no evidence that, making allowance for
differences in severity, patients cared for in hospital necessarily
fare better than those cared for at home, or that families caring
for patients at home are more stressed than the families of
patients initially cared for in hospital. Therefore, most
decisions on admission to hospital have to be based upon
practical considerations: i.e. can the patient be managed at
home with the support of the primary health care team (particularly the district nurse), taking into account the expectations of, and support available from, the rest of the family?

Immediate care

If the GP and family elect for care at home, then there are
four tasks to complete during the first visit:

1. Discussion of facts, fears and anxieties

Some people think that a stroke is an affliction of the heart,
and so a brief explanation of what a stroke is may be helpful,
stressing that it affects the brain. More important is a discussion of the likely outcome. Many people know someone

who had a stroke and died, and are convinced that the same will happen in their own case. Therefore, stressing good prognostic points, when appropriate, can be helpful. Interestingly, many patients comment that a promise to return within a few days has been their most powerful reassurance that they were not expected to die shortly!

2. Toileting arrangements

These need specific discussion with the patient and family, even if only to reassure them that it is medically safe for the patient to use the toilet or commode. Advice and help from the district nurse are frequently needed, and regular visits from her usually give an important boost to morale as well as physical support. She can quickly organize a commode, pads, etc. It is worth noting that urinary incontinence (for any reason) carries a poor prognosis for both survival and functional recovery.

3. Where the patient will be nursed

This includes considering the room (upstairs or downstairs) and whether the patient needs to stay in bed. The district nurse will often help move the patient and/or the bed. There is no good reason for excessive rest after stroke, and the patient should be encouraged to be up and about within the limits of any disability or feeling unwell.

4. Feeding and drinking

About 10% of conscious patients choke on liquids in the first 24 hours after stroke. This rarely causes serious problems, but does carry a less good prognosis for recovery. Every conscious patient should be watched drinking a glass of water: if he chokes, the patient should be cautioned against eating soups or crumbly food for 24–48 hours, and advised to start with a semi-solid diet. Many families think that the diet must be restricted or changed, and so should be reassured that normal food can be eaten (unless swallowing difficulties exist).

> One morning Mr Sweet, a 68-year-old college lecturer, suddenly developed partial paralysis on the right. He limped to his armchair and sat down. His wife called the GP who arrived to find him fully conscious, sitting in his armchair. The diagnosis of stroke was obvious and the GP soon left, thinking all would be well and saying he would arrange for a consultant to visit and advise on rehabilitation. When the consultant arrived three days later, he found Mr Sweet still sitting in the chair, afraid to move although he could do so easily. Furthermore he was soaked in urine because he thought he should not walk to the toilet. He had not eaten or slept. His wife was distraught.

The case history illustrates how easily management can fail from the very beginning. Indeed, it was perhaps the apparent mildness of the stroke that lured the GP into a false sense of security.

Each of the four points mentioned above needs active consideration, and discussion with the patient and family. Active follow-up and involvement of the district nurse is vital, particularly to avoid the family taking a mistaken course.

THE SECOND VISIT

In contrast to the first visit, which may well be a hurried emergency, the second will not, and so more time should be available, giving the GP the opportunity to set the scene for all future management. As the above case illustrates, people will often behave irrationally in an abnormal and frightening situation. Every patient being nursed at home after an acute stroke deserves an early second visit, preferably within a day or two of the stroke, and preferably by the same doctor. An early second visit allows the detection of inappropriate behaviour before too much harm is done.

Table 7.1 Principles of the management of stroke at home

---

1. Identify the problems:
   neurological deficits (see Chapter 4)
   abilities lost (see Chapter 4)
   structural obstacles in the house
   emotional and social sequelae
   family stress
2. Know likely extent of any recovery:
   how much, and how fast?
   who will do well?
3. Look for discrepancies between observed and expected function.
   'Why is the patient not doing more?'
4. Consider intervention:
   therapist(s)
   aids
   social support
   drugs
   transfer to hospital
5. Talk to the patient and family about:
   diagnosis
   prognosis
   treatment
   lifestyle
6. Reassess items 1–5 at appropriate intervals
7. Start thinking about secondary prevention (see Chapter 11)

From the second visit on, the general principles underlying effective rehabilitation are the same and are best summarized by the phrase 'Be curious – ask why'.

It is important to have an adequate knowledge of the natural history of recovery after stroke. Coupled with this it is helpful to be able to give the patient a prognosis based upon the particular features of his stroke.

RECOVERY – NATURAL HISTORY

Most patients who survive the acute illness will recover, some more than others. The prediction of who will do well is dis-

cussed later; this section considers the general rules governing
recovery as observed in groups of patients. As will be shown,
individual patients may not conform to general rules.

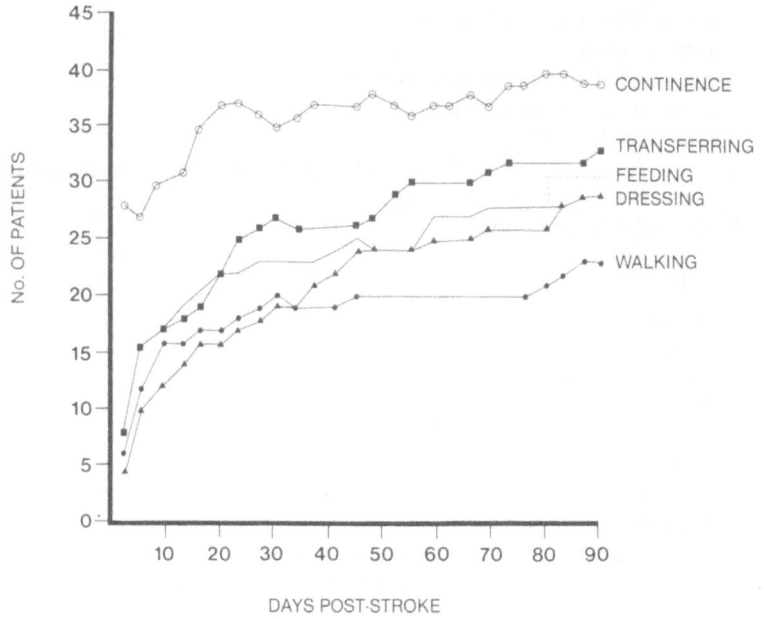

Figure 7.1   Recovery of independence (i.e. not needing help); 45
patients followed over 3 months

The fastest phase of recovery is the first few weeks. Over
50% of the total recovery made within the first 3 months will
have occurred within the first 2 weeks. This is illustrated in
Figures 7.1 and 7.2, which demonstrate recovery of ability
observed in a group of patients assessed twice a week. Figure
7.1 is based upon 45 patients from within 4 days of their
stroke, and shows the number of patients achieving complete
independence (i.e. not needing help) in a variety of abilities
over the first 3 months after stroke. It is worth noting that not
all patients lose independence; that recovery is most rapid

in the first 2 weeks; and that the curves are similar for all disabilities.

In total, 67 patients of the 100 registered in this study survived 3 months, and 47 of these were able to walk alone at 3 months. Figure 7.2 shows the percentage walking alone at each point over the first 3 months, emphasizing that 50% of those independent at 3 months were already independent by 2 weeks, but also showing that a few patients were still regaining independence at 2–3 months.

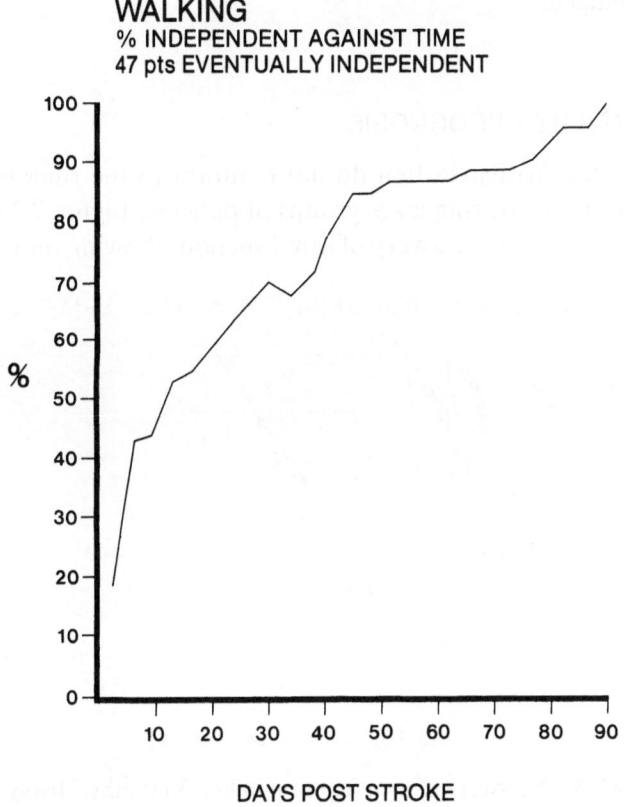

WALKING
% INDEPENDENT AGAINST TIME
47 pts EVENTUALLY INDEPENDENT

Figure 7.2 Time of achieving ability to walk unaided; 47 patients able to walk alone by 3 months

How long recovery continues is uncertain. Improvement between 3 and 6 months has been documented in many patients for most aspects of stroke loss, including memory and arm function. After 6 months it is relatively rare for dramatic recovery to be seen, but it is probable that between 5 and 10% of patients will make some significant recovery, albeit slowly and not of great extent. Two other equally important processes probably continue. First, some patients will probably improve in those areas that they have recovered – for example, dressing faster. Second, patients and families adapt their lifestyle to minimize handicap even though the neurological disability is unchanged.

RECOVERY – PROGNOSIS

Individual patients often do not conform to the rules established from studying large groups of patients. Figure 7.3 demonstrates this for recovery of arm function, showing the curves

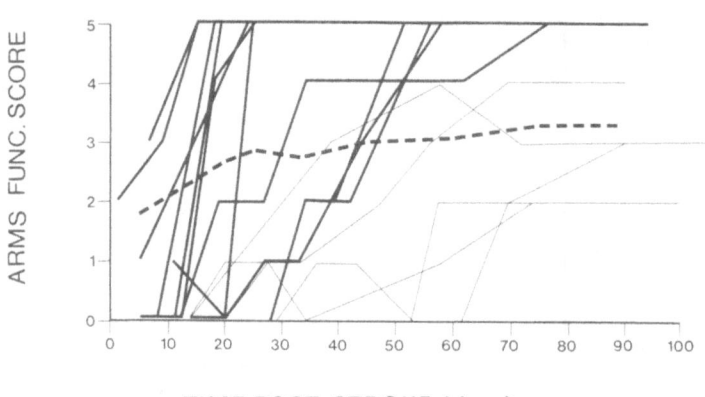

Figure 7.3   Recovery of arm function in first 3 months. Heavy lines, 11 patients making full recovery; light lines, five patients making incomplete recovery; dotted line, average score of all 56 patients studied

from 11 patients who made a full recovery and the curves from five who made a partial recovery. These 16 patients were part of a group of 56 patients. The other 30 made no recovery – 17 had useless arms, and 23 never lost function. The average arm function score of all 56 is shown by the heavy dotted line. This figure shows that virtually no patient followed the smooth path of recovery obtained by taking the average; some made a rapid and complete recovery, others a slow and incomplete one.

As a general rule, the worse someone is initially (say at 3–7 days), the worse they will be at 6 months. Figure 7.4 illustrates this for recovery of activities of daily living (ADL; e.g. dress-

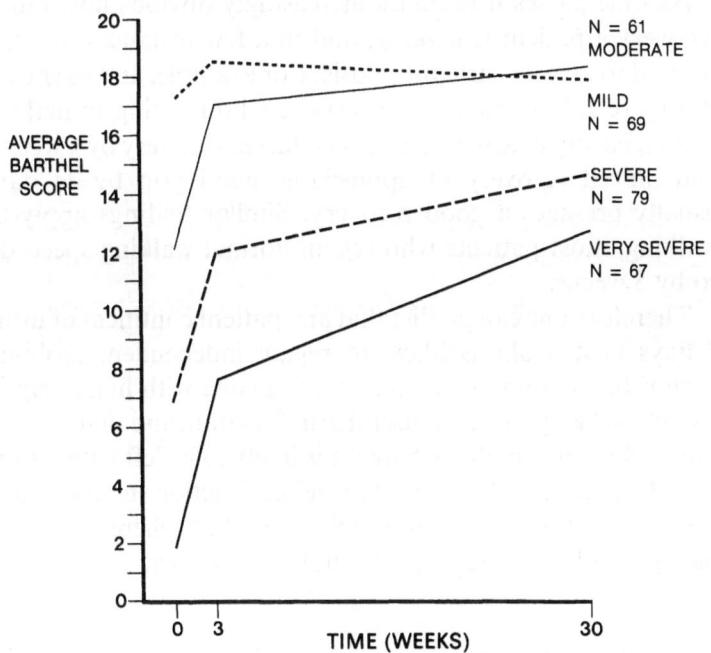

Figure 7.4 Recovery of activities of daily living (ADL). Using the Barthel ADL index (see appendix 2) – a score of 20 indicates full independence, but not necessarily normality. Patients divided into four groups according to initial disability

ing, walking). The four curves represent four groups of patients who survived 1 year, subdivided by their initial severity. Similar rules apply in other spheres such as language loss.

While it is easy to predict a good outcome for someone who is scarcely affected, it is much more difficult to identify severely disabled patients who will do better than expected. Traditional prognostic features, such as the presence of hemianopia or sensory loss, are probably primarily indicative of the general severity of the stroke rather than being of independent prognostic importance. Recent research suggests that the presence of urinary incontinence may help in giving a prognosis. It seems that people who are continent soon after stroke (say within 3 days) will make a good recovery of functional independence even if otherwise severely affected.

As time passes it becomes increasingly obvious how much recovery a patient is making, and in a few instances this can be used to give an early prognosis. For example, and as shown in Figure 7.3, it seems that everyone who is going to make a good recovery of arm function has started recovery by 4 weeks, and indeed recovery of appreciable hand grip by 24 days usually presages a good recovery. Similar findings apply to walking; most patients who regain normal walking speed do so by 5 weeks.

Therefore one can predict that any patient continent of urine 2 days post-stroke is likely to regain independent mobility even if bed-bound at the time; that anyone with hand grip at 3 weeks is likely to regain useful arm function; and that anyone not walking normally by 5 weeks is likely to be left with a slow gait. In addition, the eventual level of function in any sphere is related to the severity of initial loss in that sphere. With this background knowledge, rehabilitation can start.

FUNCTIONAL REHABILITATION

The heading is deliberately ambiguous, and is intended to include both the topic – returning patients to independence in activities of daily living – and the approach suggested – pragmatic, aimed at returning function. At present there is no evidence that a specific technique, such as the widely used Bobath approach to physiotherapy, is superior to any other technique, or to a pragmatic approach.

The vital first step in good management is to determine what the patient is actually doing or not doing, and then to compare this with what the patient should be doing, given his abilities, and with what he could be doing, given expert advice and help. In order to do this, Table 7.2 shows six areas of function which should be considered on each occasion the patient is seen during the first 12 months post-stroke.

> A 64-year-old retired warehouseman was admitted to hospital with a right hemiparesis and aphasia. He stayed 4 weeks and made a good physical recovery, had a brief home visit, and went home able to walk alone safely. His wife was told he could go upstairs 'in a few days'. Over the next 6 months he attended weekly for speech therapy and his GP called monthly to check his blood pressure. Seven months post-stroke he was able to go shopping, which entailed a long walk including steps, but still had his bed downstairs in the living room, severely restricting the family's social life. When his wife was asked why, she explained that no-one had ever said he could go upstairs, and they were afraid to do so. He was escorted up the stairs, and by that evening their life was transformed.

Despite attending a stroke unit, having a home visit and regular contact with various interested parties, rehabilitation failed this man. There was a large discrepancy between his obvious abilities – walking anywhere he wished – and his actual function, not going upstairs.

Two points need emphasis. First, one must actively inquire about the functions shown in Table 7.2. Patients will often not mention problems which, therefore, remain undetected and untreated – as in the case above. Another example is urinary incontinence, which may be first diagnosed by sitting on a wet chair. One possible solution is for a member of the primary health care team, perhaps the district nurse or health visitor,

Table 7.2

Function	Problems to consider
Cognition	Orientation, memory
	Neglect, apraxia and similar deficits
Communication	Aphasia (language loss)
	Dysarthria (slurring of speech)
Excretion	Faecal incontinence
	Urinary incontinence
	Toilet arrangements
Mobility	Moving in bed
	Getting from bed to chair
	Walking safely
	Going up and down stairs
	Going outside
Feeding	Swallowing satisfactorily
	Feeding self
Washing	Face, teeth, hands
	All over (bath/shower)
Dressing	Large items (shirt, trousers)
	Small items (buttons, laces, bra straps, etc.)

to complete a simple checklist and to leave it in the patient's house for all the other members of the team to see and amend as progress occurs.

The second point is that the patient's neurological deficits should be identified in order to alert the team to likely problems, to give the explanation for a functional loss, and to form the basis for future expectations. For example, a man with normal strength in his leg should usually be able to walk; if he is not, a reason should be sought. Also, the presence of hemianopia, for example, might alert one to difficulties with reading, or to apraxic problems, and might explain why someone is unable to dress successfully.

For each disability identified, the following questions should be asked:

1. Is it explained simply by the neurological deficits?
   If not, does the patient have other neurological deficits?
   Or is the disability exaggerated by fear or other factors?

2. Is there simple advice to alleviate matters?
3. Are matters going to improve spontaneously, and if so is further action unnecessary at present?
4. Is help needed from a district nurse, physiotherapist, occupational therapist, speech therapist, social worker, health visitor, neurologist, geriatrician or general physician?

Organizing rehabilitation

Ideally the patient should receive specialist assistance from a co-ordinated team of therapists as soon as possible; this team might constitute a district 'stroke service', probably based in the local general hospital but strongly committed to community care. At present such services do not exist in the UK. Most help is needed initially when the problems are at their most severe and complications, such as a pulled and painful shoulder, may be avoided. It is also possible that early therapy has more effect, though the effectiveness of any therapy has yet to be proved. In practice there will usually be an unavoidable delay between referral to, and arrival of, a therapist, if indeed the GP has ready access to domiciliary services outwith his primary health care team.

Two factors mitigate the problem of delay. First, much natural recovery occurs early on, rapidly resolving some difficulties. Nevertheless the patient will still have to overcome the problems until help arrives or recovery occurs. The second mitigating factor is the district nursing service. Most district nurses can see a patient within a few hours (if asked), and they are usually well experienced in the home care of acutely ill patients.

The family should be shown how to handle the patient. Particular stress should be given to techniques of moving someone in the bed, from the bed to a chair or commode, and possibly in standing and walking if appropriate. The nurse/therapist should watch the family to ensure that they are capable and safe. She could also leave suitable illustrated information leaflets, or recommend booklets for the family to borrow or buy – see appendix 3.

The difficult problem of co-ordination of health professionals remains. The number of people who may become involved with a single patient can be large. One solution is to leave a written record in the patient's home for all to see; the nursing process card used by the district nurse is suitable. The record should show the current problems (e.g. difficulty swallowing, unable to transfer); who is helping (e.g. neighbour, nurse, physiotherapist); how they may be contacted and when they will next call; the name of the GP and the surgery telephone number; and any expected action (e.g. wheelchair to arrive soon). Ultimately the GP's most important role is to organize all the services involved, ensuring that the family receive all the help they need (but not more than they can cope with).

Specialist help

Assuming that therapists cannot be organized immediately, the GP will need to start active rehabilitation for those patients left with problems at about 2 weeks, contacting therapists if needed. Where domiciliary therapy services are limited or absent, referral to an outpatient department might be necessary, but practical considerations (transport, waiting lists) often make this alternative impossible. This section considers what the more commonly available therapies might offer. It should be pointed out that different therapists in different areas may define their functions quite differently. However, there is no good reason why a physiotherapist should not cut toenails just as a district nurse often does physiotherapy.

Physiotherapy

Physiotherapists are traditionally most concerned with improving mobility. Although usually based in hospitals, there is an increasing trend towards domiciliary services being available to GPs. If this is available, it is worth asking a physiotherapist to call on any patient left with significant problems with mobility 1 or 2 weeks after the stroke. This would include any patient who has not regained his former abilities in climbing stairs and walking without assistance.

The physiotherapist should be asked to assess the patient and to give advice to the family on how to manage the problems; to give advice on the need for any aids; and to help the patient overcome particular problems. The therapist may not need to give therapy as such, but she should follow up her first visit to supervise the patient's recovery and decide whether an aid is needed, or can be taken away. Attending hospital as an out-patient is less satisfactory because physiotherapy is seen, both by the patient and by the staff, as a treatment in isolation from daily life. Furthermore, satisfactory transport to and from hospital is often extremely difficult to arrange.

Occupational therapy

Problems with dressing, cooking, feeding and other aspects of self-care more dependent upon arm function than upon mobility are usually the province of occupational therapists, who will also be concerned with neglect and other cognitive difficulties. Unfortunately, in many areas almost all this aspect of occupational therapy is carried out in hospital. Consequently it often falls to the district nurse or the physiotherapist to manage these problems at home; usually they succeed, and referral to a hospital department is not needed.

Referral to an occupational therapist should be considered for anyone left unable to care for themselves 2 months after the stroke. Earlier referral would be better, but the difficulties of out-patient attendance, coupled with the likely recovery of most patients, renders this impractical. Some of the few patients who may possibly return to work might benefit from a work assessment by an occupational therapist; this will usually require a visit to the hospital, but it is rarely needed since most stroke patients are already retired.

A second function of occupational therapists is to assess for, and authorize, the provision of aids supplied by local authorities. These therapists do visit homes, but rarely become involved in treatment or detailed assessment outside the particular requirements of their employers: Social Services.

Speech therapy

Speech therapy is the only branch of rehabilitation which has been subjected to any reasonable scientific evaluation. The results indicate that it can increase language function in some patients, but that the therapeutic aspect of the therapist's work, as delivered in the UK at least, has little or no overall effect upon a patient's language recovery. Nevertheless speech therapists do have an important role to play. First, they can identify the presence of language disturbance and discover what abilities a patient has retained, thus allowing others to communicate at an appropriate level and maximizing the patient's potential. Second, they can give advice both to the patient and his family, and to other professional staff, on the best ways to communicate.

Speech therapists can also help with problems of swallowing. Fortunately, although about 10% of conscious patients have difficulties soon after their stroke, these rarely persist.

Social workers and health visitors

These professionals should know about most local support systems for people left severely handicapped after their stroke, such as voluntary clubs and day centres. They can also give advice on benefits, retirement from work, etc. Occasionally an early referral is needed, perhaps when another family member is also disabled and needing support, but more usually referral can be delayed until the extent of any recovery is more apparent. Of course, involvement of home helps and meals-on-wheels may be necessary immediately, and can be withdrawn when no longer needed.

Talking to the family

To the GP a stroke is a relatively common *serious* disease, even though he will only see about five cases each year; to the patient and the family it is unique. An important facet of rehabilitation, which is easily overlooked, perhaps particularly when many people are involved, is the need to talk to the family. At the second and all subsequent visits or contacts, the topics below should be actively considered and discussed with the family. The emphasis will vary over time and between patients. Nevertheless, these seem to be the matters which concern people most, although they will not always be raised by patients:

(a) *Diagnosis*. Patients are often concerned as to whether there is any doubt about the diagnosis, particularly if they have not been admitted to hospital or visited by a specialist. It is anyway important to review the diagnosis over the first few weeks. The GP should specifically restate, on at least one occasion, that he is sure of the diagnosis; he may need to organize a second opinion from a consultant to reassure either himself or the family.

(b) *Activities allowed*. Most patients think they should rest, and their carers usually agree. However there is no evidence to support this, and an optimistic, active approach should be used. The patient needs to be encouraged to do as much as is possible within the limits of his disability.

Particular topics needing discussion include sexual intercourse, physical exertion and the role of stress. The patient
needs to be reassured that sexual intercourse is safe, but may
need advice on new positions or methods. Impotence is quite
common, often secondary to drugs but occasionally associated
with sensory loss affecting the penis. It should be stressed that
there is no evidence that physical exertion is harmful, and
indeed exercise should be encouraged. Quite naturally, most
patients seek an explanation for their stroke, and commonly
attribute it to 'stress', by which they may mean worry, work,
recent bereavement, etc. They then seek to minimize 'stress',
and in so doing often become bored and depressed. It should
be explained to the patient, and more importantly to his family,
that there is no good evidence to link stress with stroke, either
directly or indirectly. Therefore they may be reassured that,
for example, going on holiday and flying in commercial aircraft
pose no particular risk of a recurrent stroke.

(c) *Mood disturbance* (see also Chapter 8). Many patients are
emotionally labile soon after stroke. This is usually transient,
but the patient and the family need reassurance that control
will return. However, about one-third of survivors become
depressed – see below.

(d) *Family feelings*. A stroke may dramatically and suddenly
alter the roles of members of a family. People may need to
take on nursing, become the chief earner, act as head of the
family, or do the housework when they have not done so
previously. This change in role, coupled with natural concern
for a loved one afflicted by a serious illness, may lead to major
psychological disturbances in the family. It is important to be
aware of this, and to allow the family to express their feelings
of fear, frustration or anger. Further, no-one should forget
that some carers maltreat people disabled by stroke. Care of
the carers is covered in more detail in the next chapter.

Patients and families often forget what they are told. Rep-
etition at later visits will help, and so will simple leaflets such
as 'Twenty questions about stroke – and their answers'. The

Chest, Heart and Stroke Association (Tavistock House North, Tavistock Square, London WC1H 9JE) publish many other leaflets; some are free and the others are cheap. There are also books on stroke suitable for patients and their families – see appendix 3.

FOLLOW-UP VISITS

Most patients start recovery within 1 week (except those destined to die), and it is best to see them quite often after their stroke to check on progress; the exact frequency of visits will depend upon each patient's circumstances. At these visits one can specifically consider the need for diagnostic reappraisal and referral to therapists. The frequency of contact can then be reduced, according to need, but a formal assessment at 4–6 months is wise: most natural recovery is complete by 6 months and it is important to consider long-term needs and, of course, secondary prevention (Chapter 11).

At each visit the following questions should be asked:

1. Is the diagnosis secure?
2. Are further investigations required?
3. Is recovery progressing as expected?
4. Could the patient do more for himself than he is doing?
5. Is an aid needed, or should one be taken away?
6. Should a therapist be contacted?
7. Is the patient as socially active as before?
8. Is the patient depressed?
9. Is more (or less) support needed?
10. Is the family managing satisfactorily?
11. What about secondary prevention?

Reasons should be sought for any unexplained shortfall in recovery, physical function or social activities. In addition, progress and problems should be discussed with the patient and family, altering the balance with time but always emphasizing that activity by the patient should be encouraged.

Depression and social activities

The recognition and treatment of the emotional and social consequence of a stroke is extremely important. These aspects are sadly neglected by many hospitals, yet cause perhaps the most distress to the family. About one-third of stroke survivors are depressed, and this is particularly related to a low level of 'social and leisure' activities (i.e. activities beyond those necessary for daily living). Such patients do little beyond getting up, dressing, eating and watching TV. Whether this results from depression, or causes it, is unknown, but it is not primarily due to any physical disability.

> A retired social worker had a minor stroke with sensory symptoms only. Subjectively they never cleared, but she never had any loss of physical mobility. Nevertheless she was transformed from a very active voluntary worker, who never had a free minute, into a housebound invalid whose much more disabled companion did all the housework and shopping.

Just as the primary health care team needs to be alert to any discrepancy between neurological deficit and actual function when considering physical rehabilitation, so they should look for unexplained reduction in social activities (including work about the house). Naturally patients with severe disability will have to alter or reduce their leisure activities, but many people curtail their lives well in excess of their physical limitations. This may be due to fear, poor advice from well-meaning friends, depression, and many other reasons.

Thus the patient's pre-stroke lifestyle must be compared with his post-stroke lifestyle. A reason should be sought for any change. Some will be inevitable; a patient may no longer go to work, or might be unable to drive. However, the patient should be encouraged to return to as many activities as possible, and to take up new ones to replace any no longer possible.

Mood disorder is considered in more detail in the next chapter.

Driving

Stopping driving is a major problem to many people, and is strongly associated with depression. Any patient who has epilepsy or hemianopia as a result of his stroke should inform the licensing authorities, and will lose his licence. In our experience the response of the DVLC to stroke has not been consistent: some patients who have recovered completely within 3 months have been advised not to drive for 1 year, while other disabled drivers are allowed to do so within 6 months.

In general it is obviously sensible that someone should not drive until he can control the car safely. This may be a difficult judgement to make. The British School of Motoring, and probably other driving schools, will take disabled people out to test them in specially adapted cars. During this test the instructor will assess what adaptations are needed to a standard car, if any, and also the driver's safety. He will provide a written report with a copy for the licensing authorities. A fuller assessment is also available from the Banstead Place Mobility Centre, Park Road, Banstead, Surrey SM73 3LE; they will also give advice on what adaptations are needed to a car so that someone can drive safely. Patients aged under 65 years should consider applying for a mobility allowance, which may help them acquire a suitable car through the Motability scheme – a social worker will give advice on these and other allowances.

PATIENTS DISCHARGED FROM HOSPITAL

In practice, many patients receive their initial rehabilitation in hospital; this is particularly true of those living alone and those experiencing more severe initial disability. Over 80% of surviving patients admitted to hospital do return home, and so the primary health care team will eventually become involved in caring for most surviving patients, including many with quite severe problems.

Many patients are discharged without adequate provision

of aids or support services. The ideal, but not always practical, solution would be for the GP to visit each patient in hospital before discharge to ensure that the hospital staff are aware of the home circumstances and to prepare himself for the likely difficulties after discharge. In some areas district liaison nurses have been appointed for this specific task. In practice the GP is rarely informed of any impending discharge, and may not know until days afterwards unless he is telephoned by the house physician. The patient should be visited as soon as practical after arrival home, to try and prevent major problems developing. At that visit, and later ones, the same questions should be asked as given above.

It should never be assumed that all remediable problems have been considered by the hospital services. After discharge from the ward many patients will continue to have out-patient therapy, and most will be seen in the medical clinic at least once, which might lull the GP into a false sense of security. Unfortunately hospital staff are often unaware of home and family circumstances, and sometimes forget to identify or check on particular items, including even medical ones such as blood pressure. Therefore, for the primary health care team every patient leaving hospital should be considered as a new stroke.

In order to reduce the crisis a patient and his family often experience on leaving hospital, the GP should if possible become involved in his care while the patient is still in hospital. He will then be able to tell hospital staff about likely problems at home, and tell the family what is happening in hospital. The hospital should warn the GP not only about discharge from the ward, but also about final discharge from continuing rehabilitation, as this can cause a further crisis in the family: they suddenly realize that more recovery is not anticipated, and may feel abandoned.

AFTER RECOVERY IS OVER

Many stroke survivors lead a very restricted life. They cannot drive, cannot get onto or off the anyway infrequent buses, taxis are expensive, their spouse cannot drive, and getting into a car is difficult. In addition, they have problems getting into and out of strange buildings, and are afraid that they will not be able to manage the toilet if it is needed. They feel abnormal, and frequently are abnormal in their gait, speech and ability to use their arm. They need help.

The prevalence of stroke survivors is probably about 5–7/1000, of whom about half will have their life permanently altered by the stroke. Thus on average each GP will be caring for about eight disabled survivors and eight healthy ones – all 16 will need consideration for secondary prevention (Chapter 11).

Patients left disabled after stroke are little different from the much larger number of disabled patients, usually elderly, that every GP cares for. Although the stroke-induced problems may remain static, the patient's general health, and that of his supporters, will often change. It is also wise to reconsider the questions on page 129 and abilities on page 122 about once a year to ensure that nothing has been overlooked.

The major need for these patients is satisfactory social support, from their families, day centres, and voluntary organizations. Our own experience suggests that the major identifiable obstacle to a more fulfilling life for these patients is their inability to get from place to place. Changing our social, housing and public transport policies is probably the most effective way to improve disabled patients' quality of life: a major contribution to patients' welfare may be to draw these obstacles to the attention of politicians and planners.

PRACTICAL POINTS

Stroke presents as a sudden catastrophe which seldom requires the specialized diagnostic or treatment facilities of the hospital.

General practitioners are ideally placed to manage stroke within the context of the patient's own home and family.

Stroke patients usually require help from several members of the primary health care team, as well as other professionals including social workers, physiotherapists, etc.

The general practitioner's most important role is in problem recognition, and then knowing who can do what, and how to get them involved.

A written record in the patient's home, identifying all relevant problems and the personnel involved, may be a great help in co-ordination and ensuring that nothing is overlooked.

All concerned should always be asking themselves, 'Can the patient do more? Is his behaviour consistent with the known (neurological/medical) facts?'

8

MOOD DISORDER AFTER STROKE

Mood disorder after stroke is a common problem, and yet few clinicians have a ready answer to the management difficulties it causes. It is easy to regard it as either a natural response to stroke – and therefore likely to pass with time – or as an inherent part of the brain damage, and therefore as essentially untreatable. These attitudes produce therapeutic passivity, which does little for the doctor's enthusiasm for dealing with stroke patients, and which may lead to undertreating of a distressing and disabling condition. The purpose of this chapter is to provide an outline for the assessment and management of post-stroke mood disorder by concentrating on three main areas. Firstly, an attempt will be made to define the main clinical syndromes of mood disorder and the conditions from which they should be differentiated, paying particular attention to diagnostic problems in the elderly and brain-damaged. Secondly, some practical problems of diagnostic assessment and investigation of aetiology will be considered. Finally, an outline management plan will be suggested with some consideration of the role of drugs and of the decision about specialist referral.

MAKING THE DIAGNOSIS

Types of mood disorder

The principal features of mood disorders after stroke will be considered below, outlining the distinguishing features which suggest that they can be regarded as discrete clinical syndromes. The vague and confusing term 'depression' has been avoided, although it is frequently used by doctors and patients to describe any or all of these states.

Table 8.1   Types of mood disorder after stroke

Adjustment reactions
Depressive illness
Pathological emotionalism
Catastrophic reactions
Indifference reactions

Adjustment reactions

Stroke is sudden and unexpected, and may lead to chronic disability; both the acutely stressful event of the onset and the subsequent chronic health difficulty may be associated with emotional problems. Stress, almost by definition, leads to arousal and symptoms of tension; insomnia and restlessness are common if transient. The frustration experienced by so many patients in the early recovery phase may be seen in part as a response to enforced physical inactivity at a time of general systemic arousal. The emotions associated with stress and arousal are the natural accompaniment of the individual's disposition to flight (anxiety) or fight (irritability or aggression). In addition, there is frequently a sense of loss which leads to unhappiness or distress. It should be remembered that these emotions may be expressed indirectly; for example, fear of recurrence may lead to agoraphobia, while the desire to 'fight back' at an intangible illness may lead to irritation with a loved one. The archetypal adjustment reaction is grief, which comes on immediately after the experience of loss, and the florid symptoms of which usually resolve within weeks. Like grief, however, the range of individual emotional adjustment to stroke is great, and while the majority have re-established emotional equilibrium within 3–6 months of the traumatic experience, some patients become stuck in a state of chronic demoralization and unhappiness. A useful analogy is to think of stroke patients as grieving, but for something they have lost in themselves rather than in the outside world. Persistent or unresolved adjustment reactions can merge imperceptibly into the next condition to be considered – depressive illness.

Probably the majority of stroke patients experience some mood symptoms in the first weeks, with 30–40% having symptoms of sufficient severity to merit clinical attention. Their main importance is that they can lead to unnecessary physical and social restriction for the patient, and also impair the capacity to follow explanations or remember instructions.

Depressive illness

The clinical picture of depressive illness differs from that of the adjustment reactions in the following respects:

1. The unpleasant mood state is more invariable and unresponsive to external circumstances.
2. Biological features (insomnia, anorexia with weight loss, sexual dysfunction, etc.) are more prominent and persistent and there may be more specific symptoms such as early morning wakening or diurnal mood variation.
3. Onset may be weeks or months after the experience of stress and the disorder resolves slowly if at all.

The elderly may present a particular diagnostic problem with, for example, relatively little in the way of overt mood disturbance, but prominent biological symptoms or hypochondriasis. Because those with adjustment reactions are mainly concerned with external circumstances, and those with depressive illness are driven by an internal mood disturbance, the latter tend to be more preoccupied with pessimistic thoughts about themselves, their lives and the future in general. They are less readily reassured by pointing out that their opinions are unrealistically gloomy. Another useful clue is the presence of a family history or past personal history of psychiatric treatment for depressive illness; even if this has occurred years ago, it suggests a predisposition to the condition.

Clinically important depressive disorders are relatively common in the 'normal' elderly population, with a prevalence of about 10–15%. It is said that their prevalence in stroke patients is higher at 20–30%, with the highest risk period being in the first 6–9 months after stroke. The persistence of these disorders means that they may lead to substantial social dysfunction and handicap out of proportion to physical disability. This possibility should be entertained particularly when a patient who should be doing, or has been doing, well, plateaus or deteriorates in function. Depressive illness in the elderly can mimic dementia, and even leads to impairment on tests of orientation and memory. This diagnosis, so-called *depressive pseudodementia*, should be suspected where there are diurnal fluctuations in intellectual function, where the 'dementia' appears to have developed rapidly, or where there is a past history of depressive illness:

A 76-year-old woman was seen at home. She had suffered a left hemisphere infarct 11 months previously and had initially done well, returning from hospital after 6 weeks. Over the past 3 months she had become increasingly forgetful and restless at night. When seen, she was sitting forward in her chair clinging to her Zimmer frame but making no effort to stand. She could give no account of herself and was unable to answer orientation or memory tests. When pressed she briefly became agitated and asked to be left alone; she said there was 'no point in it' and then 'I am too old, I just want to die'. The GP's notes revealed that he had treated her for a depressive illness 10 years previously after her husband's death. She responded well to a course of antidepressants and a short spell of attendance at a psychogeriatric day hospital.

Pathological emotionalism

A tendency to be readily moved to tears, so that at times crying is unexpected and socially embarrassing, is called emotional lability, and often considered to be a feature of brain damage. However, such emotionalism should only be regarded as organically based under two circumstances:

1. When it is contextually inappropriate. Sudden or unheralded crying is a common feature of many conditions, including grief and depressive illness. Contrary to popular belief, much crying in stroke patients *is* associated with sadness, and it is only when it is not, and when its appearance is quite unprovoked, that an alternative explanation should be sought. Under these circumstances it is sometimes called 'forced' weeping.
2. When it is associated with pathological laughter, a much rarer condition usually seen only in those with pseudobulbar palsy.

There are no reliable figures on its prevalence but true organic emotionalism after stroke is probably rare, and under most circumstances weepiness in stroke patients is best thought of as a disturbance of emotional *expression* rather than one of emotional *feeling*. As such it may be understood as arising from the same causes as adjustment reactions and depressive illness, differing only in the external manifestation of the emotion. It is a common mistake to assume that tearfulness after stroke is unrelated to distress, and to miss the opportunity to discuss it as such with the patient.

Catastrophic reactions

Kurt Goldstein, who coined this term, considered it as an emotional response to tasks which are beyond the individual's capacity to fulfil. The patient is 'sullen, evasive, exhibits temper, or even becomes aggressive' in response to being pressed to perform such tasks and, because these emotions are unpleasant, the patient seeks to avoid them by withdrawal from activity or by sticking to a limited number of well-learned tasks – so-called organic over-orderliness. Despite its name then, the emotional disorder may not appear 'catastrophic', but instead presents as the all-too-familiar disinclination to participate in organized activities. It is distinguished from indifference reactions (see later) because the associated mood is truculence or aggression rather than euphoria or apathy. In one large study of brain-damaged patients about 10% were openly irritable or aggressive with their examiner, and 20% refused point blank to co-operate with some part of the assessment. These reactions are said to be commoner in those with left hemisphere damage, particularly when associated with dysphasia, and are in general thought of as organic in aetiology. They are likely to be more apparent to carers (family or professional) who often have to press the patient into some activity, and cannot be readily detected by a clinical interview unless it includes an invitation to the patient to undertake some task such as walking or attempting a test of memory.

Indifference reactions

By contrast with the above disorders, some patients exhibit a state of apathy and lack of motivation which is not associated with anxiety or distress but with a striking indifference to their circumstances. At times this response can amount to an unusual euphoria with socially inappropriate jocularity, but more commonly the picture is of an emotionally neutral disinclination to participate in activities. This latter state can be a source of considerable frustration and irritation to carers. It may be a response to an under-stimulating environment – either as a result of institutionalization or the ministrations of an over-protective relative – but is also a direct result of brain damage. At times, indifference reactions occur in association with frontal lobe damage, in which case there may be other signs such as impaired attention span or disinhibited displays of aggression or sexuality. The other site which is said to be responsible for this reaction is the non-dominant parietal lobe, in which case there is usually associated sensory neglect and perhaps complete denial of the ownership of the contralateral limbs. An interesting finding in these patients is the occasional denial of any form of disability or handicap despite the presence of severe paralysis:

> A 93-year-old lady had been in a wheelchair with a dense left hemiplegia ever since her stroke 6 months previously. Towards the end of a long interview, during which she had discussed her unhappiness at her condition, she asked if she could be found a little job helping an old person with their housework as a way of cheering herself up. When asked how she could do that she said she felt sure that she would be well enough 'in a few days' if only the nurses would let her do more now.

Denial of illness is not itself very common, but the phenomena with which it is associated, such as sensory or visual neglect, are found in about 50% of right hemisphere stroke patients. Usually only those with extensive parietal lobe damage have such signs, and even then they usually resolve in a few weeks. Their importance is that they are associated with a poor long-term functional outcome, perhaps because of the degree of damage required for their emergence, or perhaps because they are such disabling impairments *per se*.

Differential diagnosis

A number of primarily physical disorders can mimic mood disorder, and should be considered even when the presenting complaint of the patient or carer is the latter. These disorders fall into two groups:

1. Cognitive problems which mimic the intellectual problems which may accompany depression in the elderly, and which may themselves be associated with anxiety due to poor performance and poor comprehension.
2. Medical problems which mimic the biological symptoms of depression and the associated lassitude, slowing, apathy and withdrawal.

Cognitive problems after stroke are sufficiently common and important that they are worth looking for in every patient who is having emotional or behavioural difficulties. A useful screening test is the Mini Mental State Examination (appendix 2) which can be readily completed by any visiting professional in 5–10 minutes. It provides pointers to difficulties with language, design copying (non-dominant parietal lesions) and memory, as well as giving a global score which is a simple guide to intellectual impairment (the cut-off score is 24 or below). Psychological testing is rarely included in the medical examination in hospital or general practice, and yet a simple, quick and acceptable test such as this may provide useful and unexpected information on the presence or absence of organic intellectual impairment.

> A 59-year-old Polish woman suffered an embolic brainstem stroke due to rheumatic mitral valve disease. She gradually thereafter became withdrawn, neglected herself, appeared uninterested in visitors and developed urinary incontinence. When seen 3 months after her stroke she appeared indifferent to her surroundings and unwilling to be interviewed. Her age and the nature of the stroke made the hospital diagnosis of 'dementia' unlikely, and indeed with gentle persistence she scored 26 on the Mini Mental State. A provisional diagnosis of depressive illness was made and she eventually responded well to a course of tricyclic antidepressants.

General medical problems may also lead to changes in mental state. Patients with cerebral damage respond differently to many drugs, a fact which is easy to overlook when the drug was being prescribed before the stroke. In particular, those drugs which act on the nervous system (e.g. hypnotics, antidepressants and antiparkinsonian agents) may produce sedation or agitation after stroke even if the dosage is the same as it was beforehand. Many hypotensive drugs cause lethargy and even depressive illness.

Investigation of acute or chronic confusional states in the elderly is a subject beyond the scope of this book, but should not be neglected simply because the patient has had a stroke.

THE CLINICAL ASSESSMENT

Having outlined the main mood disorders which may be encountered after stroke, and important conditions from which they should be differentiated, the next question is: what should the general practitioner undertake in the way of clinical assessment of mood disorder in stroke patients? Family doctors are always being exhorted to screen their patients for this or that condition, but they are only likely to respond if there is a feasible means for them to do so within the framework of their routine work, and if by so doing the patients can be helped. Some practical suggestions are outlined below.

Detecting mood disorder

The decisions to be made can be summarized by answering the questions:

1. How actively should mood disorder be sought in those who do not complain of it openly?
2. If mood disorder is to be actively sought, when is the best time to look?

Almost every patient after stroke is fearful – of recurrence, physical disability, or dependence. Also for many elderly people, stroke (as a disease affecting the brain) raises the spectre of dementia. Actively pursuing these anxieties, and asking about others, is a great benefit to people, not because it allows bland reassurance but because a doctor who shows willingness to face realistic emotional concerns is more likely to be trusted and listened to on other matters:

A woman of 50 suffered a cerebral haemorrhage which fortunately left her with little physical disability. After normal angiography she was discharged with the reassurance that nothing more was to be done. At interview a month later she initially denied problems, but when asked specifically about fears of recurrence she broke down and admitted that she was terrified of being left alone. She went on to say that she expected a recurrence at any moment because stroke was 'in the family'. It transpired that her son had developed a cerebral abscess 6 years previously, and she was unaware that this was a different condition.

If these problems are raised early it may help to encourage active rehabilitation in the first weeks. In later weeks depressive symptoms should be sought, particularly in those with many physical complaints or those who are doing unexpectedly badly in terms of rehabilitation. Again a useful way in may be to ask about previous experiences with other stroke patients:

A man of 62 was seen 6 months after a left hemisphere infarct which had left him with a mild hemiparesis and word-finding difficulty. He had not left the house unaccompanied since the stroke, and was avoiding socializing. When asked directly, it emerged that his grandmother had lived with him for 10 years following a stroke and had clearly suffered from senile dementia before her death. He had interpreted his dysphasia as an indication that the same fate awaited him.

Because mood disorder can be context-related, professionals other than the GP may be better placed to notice it. Discrepancies between reports from visiting nurses, or occupational or physiotherapists, and observations made in a clinical interview, are not always due to variations in reporting. They are more likely to be due to the different settings in which the patient is seen and can, therefore, be a useful diagnostic guide.

Assessing the aetiology

A common pitfall is to conclude that problems complained of *after* a stroke are necessarily the *result* of a stroke. It cannot be emphasized too strongly that an individual's personality and social circumstances are important determinants of outcome – particularly long-term psychological outcome – after stroke:

> A man of 48 was referred for a psychiatric opinion because of aggressive behaviour after a stroke and because he had made sexual advances to his daughter's schoolfriend. At interview he denied both problems and expressed considerable resentment at the referral. When his wife was seen alone, she confessed that he had been cautioned by the police on one occasion for exposing himself before the stroke, and that throughout their marriage he had been prone to alcohol abuse and violence. The main change was that his enforced unemployment was keeping him at home more.

This case illustrates the interplay of organic and social factors in aetiology and the value of seeing patient and carer separately at times. On the other hand, seeing both together may highlight discrepancies in attitude or behaviour which can explain frustration, irritability or unhappiness:

> A 53-year-old man appeared anxious and tearful 3 months after a stroke. No clear reason was apparent, but when he was seen with his wife she constantly interrupted, answered questions for him and treated him like a child. When this was pointed out it emerged that she followed him everywhere for fear of recurrence, even knocking on the toilet door every few seconds to make sure he was alive. He had not wished to criticize her to the doctor because of her obvious concern for him.

It should be remembered that hostility or overprotectiveness are not attitudes found only in families; the staff of nursing homes, wardens, and even doctors and nurses are not immune. Again the theme is that the place and company in which a patient exhibits mood disorder are important clues to its aetiology. As far as assessing the contribution of brain damage goes, the difficulty is that because all stroke patients are damaged to some extent it is tempting either to look past it for psychosocial problems in those with mood disorder, or to attribute all mood disorder to brain damage in a blanket way.

There is only a weak correlation between degree of intellectual impairment after stroke and subsequent mood disorder, so in this sense a 'severe' stroke physically may not be a 'severe' one mentally. There is, however, evidence that the *location* of the lesion can be influential. Frontal lesions are more commonly associated with disinhibition and aggression, and non-dominant hemisphere lesions with the syndrome of indifference and denial of deficit. Depressive illness has usually been considered as being provoked in a non-specific way by brain damage, but recently claims have been made that it is associated with left hemisphere lesions and particularly more anteriorly placed ones.

ASPECTS OF MANAGEMENT

Considerable emphasis has already been laid in this and other chapters on the value of open discussions with patient and carer. Three areas will be covered in this section: advice for carers on the management of irritability; the place of drugs in treatment; and the indications for specialist referral.

Irritability and the carer

As mentioned above, irritability is a common feature of catastrophic reactions and is therefore likely to arise when the patient has to *do* something. In a typical situation the patient has to get ready to go out or undertake some rehabilitation task such as walking exercises. He is disinclined to do so but the task is important. As pressure is applied he becomes more truculent, but what can the carer do? Insistence only increases irritation on both sides, and perhaps produces an aggressive outburst. If the task has not been completed it must be either shelved or tackled again, with the risk of the whole cycle being repeated. Advice is difficult. Either the carer walks away and 'gives in', or insists and risks provoking even more trouble.

Using the model of the catastrophic reaction reminds one that the patient's behaviour is due to being presented with a task beyond his capacity rather than simply to intransigence. It may help to break the task down into smaller units, each of which can be tackled as an independent job. For the carer, having something else to do at the same time can be a good idea, as it helps to structure the repetitive process of presenting a task and waiting until it is assimilated before moving onto the next:

A severely impaired stroke patient started shouting the moment the nurse arrived to help wash or dress him. Ignoring the shouting sometimes worked, but at other times it led to aggressive behaviour in which he would lash out and strike the nurse. By breaking down the procedure into a large number of small steps the additional time taken was only 15 minutes, but there were no further violent outbursts. Typical steps were – place flannel and soap by side and walk away, put socks by feet and wait, put on shirt and leave buttons. Between each step a pause was built in, e.g. leave room to fetch towel, sit in chair and chat about news.

This process allows a measured degree of insistence on completion of small tasks without confrontation blowing up to unmanageable proportions. It sounds easy, but many carers only learn it by being taught during direct participation. A useful approach is to arrange for a nurse to visit for a short time with the aim of teaching rather than taking over the task.

Drug treatments

Despite the frequency of mood disorder after stroke, there is evidence that GPs do not prescribe antidepressants very often. One reason may be that depression is not regarded as appropriately treated by drugs and undoubtedly there is also widespread concern about side-effects of tricyclic antidepressants in the elderly and brain-damaged. Sedation, confusion and hypotension are well known problems and are likely to occur in the elderly even at orthodox therapeutic dosage. There are two ways round this problem:

1. Use drugs with relatively few side-effects, such as mianserin or dothiepin;
2. Start at low daily dosage, e.g. dothiepin 25 mg, mianserin 10 mg, and increase by increments of the same order, every 3–4 days.

With either approach it is important not to give up too soon. Once the decision has been made to undertake a trial of antidepressants, then the best plan is to prescribe the chosen drug at its maximum tolerated dosage for 3–4 weeks at least. Many older patients cannot tolerate more than 50–75 mg per day of a standard tricyclic, but individual tolerance varies greatly, and some can take 'normal' adult doses, e.g. dothiepin 150 mg, or mianserin 90–120 mg per day. If there is no benefit then try a different drug, again at maximum tolerated dosage for a month. Only then is it reasonable to conclude that a full trial of medication has failed. Common errors are to leave a drug at an ineffective dosage, to persist for months with a drug which is not working without trying an alternative, or to abandon drugs as ineffective when neither dosage nor drug type has been modified to assess response to a different regimen.

Stroke patients – particularly the elderly – are also more sensitive to the effects of other psychotropic medication. Long half-life benzodiazepine hypnotics (nitrazepam, flurazepam) are especially likely to cause trouble with daytime sedation or confusion, but if possible all hypnotics and daytime tranquillizers should be avoided completely. A useful drug if restlessness or agitation is a major problem is thioridazine, a phenothiazine with relatively little in the way of parkinsonian or hypotensive side-effects. A low starting dose, e.g. 10 mg t.d.s., can be gradually incremented, if necessary, without producing undue sedation to the maximum tolerated dosage – usually 100–150 mg per day.

Referral to other agencies

The usual indications for specialist referral apply – help with diagnostic problems, advice over medical treatment, or the provision of services not otherwise available to the general practitioner. To take the last point first, frequently the most useful service which may be available is day-place assessment in a psychogeriatric or geriatric day hospital, or a local authority day centre. This will allow the influence of environment on mood and behaviour to be assessed, while day hospitals also allow manipulation of drug regimens, physical investigation and closer diagnostic assessment. Where mood disorder is concerned, the main diagnostic question is whether poor function (physical, social or intellectual) might be due to an atypically presenting depressive illness. Partly the answer to this question may be provided by response to tricyclics, and therefore another indication for referral is difficulty with drug treatment at home. Hospitals have the advantage of supervising compliance as well as the possibility of using more potent drugs with blood-level monitoring. Because of the complicated interplay of social and organic factors in aetiology, and the frequent coexistence of physical and psychiatric pathology, it is individual circumstances which will determine whether medical or psychiatric referral is more important. A major deciding factor is mobility, as most psychiatric facilities are poorly equipped to deal with those who are not independent in walking. Another difficulty is lack of communication between these essentially hospital-based facilities and the primary health care team. In many places, geriatricians and psychiatrists will undertake domiciliary assessment of cases like these; early use of such a service, and joint discussion of the opinion obtained, can improve subsequent care by establishing a co-ordinated management plan.

PRACTICAL POINTS

Ask all patients directly at an early visit regarding their concern about recurrence, disability and dementia. Ask about their experience of others who have had strokes.

Ask carer and visiting professionals about observable anxiety, tearfulness, withdrawal, apathy or irritability.

Consider depressive illness in patients who function surprisingly poorly, or deteriorate after early progress, and in those with unexplained physical symptoms.

Suspect depressive pseudodementia if intellectual deterioration is rapid, 'dementia' seems to fluctuate markedly, or there is a past history of depressive illness.

Check that the onset of mood disorder is really related to the stroke. Ask about antecedent stress such as bereavement or difficulties in relationship with the carer. See the patient and carer separately and together on different occasions, to yield useful information on relationships at home.

The circumstances surrounding displays of irritable or aggressive behaviour – particularly whether they are related to specific people or to tasks – will help determine whether the problems are organic or due to relationship difficulties. Always ask the emotionally labile patient why he or she is crying.

Adjustment reactions are best dealt with by early discussion of worries and actively bringing up likely anxieties. Avoid unfounded reassurance, acknowledge realistic worries. Explain and check that the explanation has been understood.

Advise carers about 'breaking up' tasks into smaller units and avoiding confrontation when aggression is a problem.

A change of environment by referral to a day centre, or for day hospital attendance, is a useful diagnostic test, may provide clues to future management at home, and can be a therapeutic exercise in itself.

If antidepressants are used, start with low doses and build up gradually to maximum tolerated dosage. Be prepared to try a second drug if the first fails. Consider referral if the indications for drugs seem good but the response is poor.

9

SUPPORTING THE CARERS OF STROKE PATIENTS

Stroke is a family illness; it causes a dramatic change and challenge to the lifestyles both of patients and their carers. Among all the groups who contribute to recovery after stroke, family and friends are generally the people most directly involved in looking after the patients. The response to the stroke of the family and main supporters is a significant influence on the attitude of patients to the illness; the response of patients to rehabilitation services; and probably the patients' rate of recovery.

The ability of the family to provide nursing care is usually the most significant factor influencing the general practitioner's decision to admit the patient to hospital, while the willingness and ability of carers to respond to problems of mobility, communication, money or domestic difficulties may determine whether the patient can remain at, or return, home. When the patient is living at home, carers have an important influence on the use of, and satisfaction with, services. They have a more general impact on recovery through their involvement in rehabilitation and, in their everyday lives, by influencing what stroke patients do for themselves.

The ways in which carers may support the recovery of patients, and how this can be reinforced by general practitioners, have been the subject of other chapters. Clearly, consideration of the carers' capacity or ability to care goes together with thinking about the impact of stroke on the carer.

This chapter concentrates on the health and quality of life of the carers and discusses how the general practitioner, with others in the primary health care team, can maintain or improve this. It aims, in particular, to identify major worries or difficulties faced by carers following the stroke. In other chapters, reference has been made to the need for patients and carers to be well informed about diagnosis, prognosis and management of the stroke. It has been indicated that the general practitioner often needs to raise issues himself – about behavioural and mood disturbance, or reduced social contacts – which patients and families may consider either trivial or embarrassing. This skilled identification of problems and gaps in information demands that the primary health care team has a familiarity with home relationships and domestic circumstances.

The knowledge, experience, health and material resources of carers vary as much as those of the general population, so that different strategies are required to meet the needs of different groups. In order to give some perspective and priority to the issues this chapter will draw upon some results from surveys of the carers of stroke patients in Greenwich and Oxfordshire. It looks at their main worries at different stages after the stroke, at current gaps in information, and at the effects of the stroke on carers and their families. General practitioners have continuing responsibilities and, therefore, longer-term perspectives than most hospital doctors. So this chapter looks in particular at the needs for longer-term support for caring in the community.

WHO ARE THE CARERS?

More than 1¼ million people in Britain today are caring for disabled or elderly relatives. About three-quarters of the carers of stroke survivors are women, overwhelmingly wives and daughters. Altogether about 90% of carers are family members, of whom about half are spouses and a quarter children of the stroke patient. These proportions depend upon the age of the patients, simply because fewer older patients have living spouses. The study of patients in Greenwich was limited to people aged 60 or over, compared with all ages in the Oxfordshire study. The consequent differences in the relationship of carers to the patients is shown in Table 9.1.

Table 9.1   Relationship of carers to patients (percentages)

	Greenwich (n = 147)	Oxfordshire (n = 94)
Wife	24	43
Husband	10	16
Daughter	27	20
Son	17	5
Other relative	10	5
Other	12	11

When the patient lives together with others, then someone from the household is nearly always the principal carer, and even when patients live alone they usually readily identify a main source of help and support, most often a son or daughter. About 10% of all stroke patients have no strong family ties or reliable source of help, and this group may be better known to general practitioners since they have to rely more often on statutory services.

About five out of every six carers are married, a similar proportion have children, and more than a third are employed at the time of stroke. But the health of many carers is less than good; half or more have some long-standing illness or health problem which is likely to affect their ability to cope with some of the demands of the patient or the illness. In some cases the stroke survivor has been the main supporter of the carer before the stroke. More often, though, the main carer has been providing some level of help and support to the patient before the stroke.

It is not only the tasks or demands of caring which may change with the onset of a stroke, but also the rewards. The carers' optimism and energy, which affect their capacity for caring, change over the course of recovery, and as they adjust to living with the consequences of the stroke. This all requires continuing assessment of the costs and benefits from the carers' perspective.

Becoming a carer

During the acute phase of stroke there is usually a pulling together of family and friends. However, the main candidate as carer is soon identified and, as it becomes clear that the patient will survive, the network of supporters is recast so that this single individual takes most of the responsibility for doing or organizing the necessary help and support. It is unusual to have more than one family member doing a major part of the job of caring. As time goes by the priorities and concerns of the main carer change in response to the needs and behaviour of the patient, and to the availability of support from elsewhere, including the health services. As a principal member of the 'team' caring for the patient, the family carer needs consistent and predictable support from other members. The aim should be to make the job of caring as satisfying as possible.

Contacts with the general practitioner

In city areas, especially in London, many patients go directly to hospital without contacting their doctor. The proportion of cases in Greenwich and Oxfordshire in which the patient's general practitioner was called is shown in Table 9.2.

Table 9.2 Coming into medical care: series of stroke patients who survived to at least 3 weeks after the stroke (percentages)

	Greenwich (n = 153)	Oxfordshire (n = 131)
Contacted a general practitioner	57	92
Went direct to casualty	38	5
In hospital at time of stroke	5	3

When patients go direct to hospital the general practitioner may not be aware of the family coping with a crisis until after the patient's discharge from hospital; and the carers consequently may receive little support from the primary care team. In the London borough of Greenwich only a quarter of the carers said they had had any helpful advice from the patient's general practitioner during the first 6 months after the stroke. In contrast, half of the supporters of patients in Oxfordshire described helpful contact with the general practitioner within the first 4 weeks of the stroke.

What makes a contact helpful? In large measure the supporters' criteria are personal rather than directly medical, and boil down to feeling that the doctor shows a *caring interest*. Among those who do not receive a visit from their long-standing general practitioner, there is a feeling of neglect. The wife of a patient home after 1 week in hospital commented:

> I would have thought someone would have made a house call – to show some caring and some help. If I hadn't gone to the doctor I don't think he would have called. There is no real consolidated help.

Of course, the general practitioner may not have known that the patient had had a stroke unless the discharge letter had arrived.

Where supporters do have contact with their general prac-

titioner in the first weeks the communication may not be
viewed as adequate:

> He just said it was a stroke. He never came back to check or
> anything.

> Spoke on phone, but only to be told that mother had had a stroke.

The carers sometimes felt that, after the diagnosis, they were
left with instructions, essentially to carry on alone:

> Explained it was a stroke. Found I was unemployed and that was
> it. It was do this, do that for him.

> He's always loath to come out. He knows what Joe is like. But he
> tells me what we must do, as if we should do it. I've told him I
> can't manage but he continues to say the same.

The difference between these comments and those of the people
who found contact with the general practitioner helpful
appears to be related mostly to the continuity of support
offered by the doctor. It seems that the key to helpful support
is reassurance that the situation is under control, and that the
doctor is going to be available when needed:

> He monitored things. He brought me in on it. Talked to me like
> a professional.

> I went down to the surgery and I saw him. He talked to me about
> George. It was reassuring but he didn't actually give me advice.
> It was more 'I'm here if you need me' sort of thing.

> She explained what a stroke was. I asked her what to do if she
> had another one – should I call 999 or call the clinic; I worried
> about that. She said call the surgery and the doctor would get
> there immediately. She said there wasn't usually any need for an
> ambulance in stroke cases. That eased my mind.

CONCERNS AND ANXIETIES

The first weeks

In the first weeks after the stroke the carers are usually more
concerned about the illness and future prospects than are

the patients, who are often confused and bewildered by the experience. For carers these first few weeks are a time of anxiety, as are other periods of major transition or change; from hospital to home, and on discharge from active rehabilitation. At different stages in the process of recovery the priorities and concerns of the carers are different, and generally not the same as the patients'.

In the early phase supporters self-evidently want to have a clear diagnosis and usually prefer an honest, even if poor, prognosis:

> The GP is a friend. We've met for drinks and he's told me what's what. ... Everyone else makes polite noises and says 'if he rests', and 'only time will tell'. It makes me sick.

Carers nearly always want the patient to return to or remain at home, but in the first weeks there is a lot of uncertainty about how fit the patient will be to come home. This leads to a multitude of concerns and worries, about the 'who' and the 'how' of caring for someone whose health and mental state is seen to be unpredictable:

> I'm worried about her financially. I'm worried about whether she's going to be able to cope physically and look after the dog. How far she's going to become depressed about the further limitations on her life. I'm worried about the possibility of a further stroke that might disable her more. I'm as worried as I can be about every part of her life. I think it's all going to be extremely difficult, but I try not to let her see I'm worried because she is worried enough herself about how she's going to manage. One of the great sources of depression has been 'I don't want to go into a home, be a vegetable' – she's absolutely determined not to go into a home. Her GP said some time ago she should be thinking about sheltered accommodation, but she won't consider it.

The lists of concerns about how the stroke survivor will cope are complemented by a similarly extensive repertoire of questions about how the supporter will cope. Carers need reassurance that although they are important members of the caring team there are other players. It appears to many that it is either their help or no-one's; the future is with them alone in

the community, or else the patient will be left with no option
except residential care:

> I'm scared they are going to send him home before he's well
> enough. They send people out that look worse than him. I couldn't
> give up my job to look after him, I'd go round the bend. But I'd
> never leave him on his own. I just wish he had someone else that
> could share the burden with me. I'm the only one left. I wish I
> knew he was being looked after and that. I'd hate him to go into
> a home.

When the patient is in hospital, and appears to be recovering
slowly, the prospect of the patient coming home may generate
not only uncertainty but despondency. How will the supporter
cope with the bathing, lifting, shopping and other physical
work that must be done? Few carers received advice about
methods of lifting or physically supporting the patient. Who
will make sure there is a new stair rail, toilet seat or possibly
a phone fitted? And who will be there when they cannot?

In these early weeks following the stroke carers need several
different sorts of support:

1. *practical* – to organize help, reconsider housing, sort out
   pensions, learn skills of rehabilitation;
2. *explanation* – about the cause of the stroke, treatment,
   prevention of a further episode, about the patient's impairments, reasonable short-term goals and realistic expectations for longer-term recovery; and
3. *social* – reassurance that other help is available, listening
   to the carer's problems. Consideration of the impact on the
   carer and the family, preparing the carer for mood changes
   in the patient, strain on personal relationships, and domestic role changes.

The next few months

Over the 6 months following stroke most patients die or return
home – both outcomes should involve preparation and support
for the carer. When the patient is back in the community the

most common criticism of general practitioners is simply that they show a lack of interest – they have not been in touch or visited to see how things are. In general, however, observations about failures in the health and social services are directed primarily to the responsibilities of the latter – particularly over housing, holidays for the patient and carer, and pension, heating and other allowances. Supporters complain little about help with practical jobs such as helping the patient on the toilet, dressing or shopping, in part because some receive help with these jobs and in part because, even where there are difficulties, it is usually accepted that this is just something one does to help.

By the middle of the first year after stroke the single most common source of upset to the carers is change in the patient's mood or personality:

> The mental frustration part of it, the physical problems don't upset me at all. I find it hard to take the mental change in him.

> The confusion in his mind. I could take the disability if his mind was alright.

> I don't really know. I can't express it … very difficult, cussedness, I suppose really. He can be very cussed at times, this is when he does cause me stress, when he's awkward.

> He used to be a kind and loving man. He's so different but he doesn't know it. I don't like having people here now because of the way he is. That upsets me. He behaves badly.

The majority of patients may be only dimly aware of the changes in their own character. It is of paramount importance to realize that from the carers' point of view such changes often cause greater distress and handicap than the difficulties posed by the physical disabilities of the patient. The low morale of many patients is another major source of distress to carers:

> To see him like he is and to see how depressed and miserable he is.

This is part of the more general observation that it is upsetting to see just how dependent one's spouse or parent has become. Many carers find it difficult to adjust to this:

I think seeing her helpless. She was very very independent-spirited, and for her to be like that was what crushed her at the beginning.

Depression and dependency among patients have important effects on the carers' relationship with the patients and on their social life. Limitation of their social activities is, at this stage, the most upsetting aspect of the illness for about one in five carers:

I do miss going out together like we used to. I do get a bit depressed over that.

Not being able to go out and do things together. This is what we are missing. We can only get out if my daughter comes.

Being tied to the house itself because that's where she is.

It's always on your mind sort of thing. She's always saying she gets lonely. I always feel when I go out, I shouldn't be going because she can't go out.

For some supporters the isolation is also a problem, feeling not only that they should not leave the stroke patients on their own, but that they have been left alone to manage:

Being left to get on with it with no help whatsoever. I feel someone should be coming to see me, to see if I'm doing it right. I feel somebody should have been.

The remainder of the family don't bother, don't take their share. She's got a big family. It upsets her as well.

Altogether about one-third of carers feel that they should be receiving some more help and support from family and friends, especially from the patients' children. A similar proportion, 30%, feel there should be more help available from the health and social services.

The longer term

The problem of coping with changes in the patient's personality or mood persists as a major cause of distress over the first and subsequent years following the stroke. It is not a problem with which supporters receive much help, and among the families of younger patients it is often the major cause of deterioration in their quality of life. During this first year of coping with the consequences of stroke, the general practitioner must consider the morale of the carer. A framework should be provided within which carers can, if they wish, vent their fears, frustrations and feelings about the patients. To maintain a positive attitude to caring it may be useful to organize 'time-off' for the carer, or to suggest participation in a carer's support group which can offer sharing of knowledge, skills and support.

It appears that towards the end of the period of noticeable recovery, say a year or more following the stroke, many supporters are disappointed. They revise their expectations for recovery throughout the process and, realistically, after a year very few expect any further improvements. It is the carers' *perception* of the disability and handicap which most influences their response to the stroke and, viewing improvement as ended, the lack of physical recovery may then assume more importance. The patient's continuing helplessness becomes a major cause of distress to carers:

> His disability, that he can't do anything. Nobody likes to feel they're relying on other people all the time.

> I don't like to see her like it and knowing that she can't cope with life by herself.

Patients who are still speech-impaired after a year or more cause particular concern:

> His speech, if you can converse you're happy in what you are doing. If he could only get his speech back and I could understand him more.

About a third of all carers say the patient has long-term problems in communication, particularly with remembering and expressing what he or she wants to say. This may reflect some confounding of intellectual with speech problems; it is often difficult for carers (and others) to know how much the patient understands.

The carers of patients with communication problems may be particularly receptive at this stage to advice and new ideas. In general, information on causes, consequences and coping with symptoms should be available at the time when an issue is of most concern to the carer. Personal contact may be supplemented by leaving publications from the Chest, Heart and Stroke Association with the carers (see appendix 3).

This stage towards the end of visible recovery should be a time for review, to consider again the help that carers need or are willing to accept, and to consider how the carers can help to maintain the patients' level of independence. It is important to discuss what level of independence patients and carers would prefer the patient to have; 'over-protective' may be an inappropriate label for what is a good balance of costs and benefits for the patient and carer involved.

GAPS IN INFORMATION

Many carers feel that they have been badly prepared for the consequences of the stroke, and that they lack information for coping with patients at home. With regard to the stroke there is a persistent question about its cause and what can be done to prevent another one. What role, for example, might stress in home or family relationships play? And are there any signs that warn of recurrence? It is difficult for carers without previous experience of the illness to know what questions to ask. Furthermore, they tend to emphasize their own independence and self-sufficiency, and are reluctant to ask for help and information. It is only with hindsight that carers realize they were not well prepared. As their expectations of recovery and relief recede, so too does their satisfaction with the information they have received.

The general practitioner and the community services are generally more likely than hospital or rehabilitation services

Table 9.3 Help, advice, and instruction received by carers in the 9 months after the stroke (percentage)

	Hospital doctor (n=85)	Hospital nurse (n=85)	Physio-therapist or occupational therapist (n=94)	Speech therapist (n=94)	GP (n=95)	District nurse or health visitor (n=95)	Social worker (n=95)
No contact	62	69	78	93	46	70	57
Contact but not helpful	26	21	6	2	30	12	16
Helpful	12	10	16	5	24	18	27

to have contact with the carers. Table 9.3 shows that this is the case in the Greenwich study, and that these services are a source of helpful advice, but it also indicates that there are many lost opportunities for providing advice and information.

In the series of carers from Greenwich, seen in the second year after a stroke, less than one-third described themselves as well prepared with advice and information for the problems they had to face. Only one in five carers said they had seen their own general practitioner to discuss any difficulties caused by the stroke. General practitioners may be good listeners but they, or someone like the district nurse or social worker, must also be good at providing unsolicited information about:

Expectations

> Nobody told me a thing about it, what to expect and what to do about it. Her diet. The things you get told are by people who've had people with strokes. It's the home help that's told us about things like getting the bed higher and the toilet seat.

> They don't tell you anything, what it's like, what to expect. They don't even tell you what's wrong. I should have expected a social worker to make enquiries about how we're coping. They're not a bit helpful.

On getting help

> You should be able to get on to somebody and find out what you should do. You get no answers from the doctor. There should be somewhere you could go. Someone that the doctor could say 'if you need help phone this number'.

> I'd like to have known a lot more about how to use the medical and social facilities that there are.

> I could have done with more information in regard to what people to contact, where I could get other help. I've had to dig and find out for myself.

And finally on the *psychosocial aspects*:

> I would have liked things explained to me a bit. He was sent home and I was told he might get a bit depressed. They said he was quite self-sufficient. My goodness – I was not prepared for it.

I think it would have been nice to have known that she was going to change so completely, to a miserable old lady.

IMPACT OF STROKE ON CARERS

In the longer term, the psychosocial sequelae of stroke – especially the patients' mood, behaviour and attitudes – seem to exact a greater toll on the carers than do the physical impairments. The consequences of the stroke for the lives of the carers are made up of several related strands – social, economic, physical and psychological. Carers suffer many of the same handicaps as patients; in particular they view the stroke as having restricted their lives:

> I cannot go out anywhere; I don't go to anything. I've had to cancel appointments because I couldn't keep them: dental appointments, hairdressing, so many things.

> Sometimes I'd like to go out somewhere, but I can't go because I don't like to leave her. I feel guilty I can go out and she can't.

The majority of carers who live with stroke patients worry about leaving them on their own. In many cases the general practitioner should be able to reassure the patient and carer that there is usually no good reason for this constant watchfulness. A significant proportion of carers view themselves as tied to the patients' home, trapped by the patients' needs, with little or no time for themselves:

> The fact that I've got all the work to do. I've got everything on my shoulders. I can't call my life my own now. My life's dictated from the time I get up to the time I go to bed.

> My life's just sitting here waiting to go down there. That's all.

Altogether, more than half of all carers view their social lives as restricted by the stroke, one-fifth as being 'severely restricted'. This has implications for the opportunities that carers have to receive support from others, as well as for the enjoyment of relief from caring:

> It's just stopped our normal life. You can't go anywhere; you can't have any holidays.

The loss of companionship, along with disruption of social and leisure activities, is a major reason for loss of enjoyment in life.

Caring for the stroke patient commonly, in about one in three cases, results in problems for other members of the carer's family – especially for the children, who have less of their parents' time. The demands of caring may cause friction in the carer's own family, usually with the spouse, but deterioration in this relationship is likely to be less marked than in that of the carer and the patient. Among the carers in Greenwich, the proportion who described their relationship with the patients as 'very happy' fell from a comfortable majority before the stroke to a minority by 1 year after the stroke. A major contribution of the primary health care team, which will be the same for the patient and their carer in half the cases, is to promote communication – to get over mutual incomprehension and to help patient and carer to understand the problems that each faces. Poor communication may lead to unrealistic expectations of each other, and so to either over-protectiveness or a failure to give help when the patient needs it. Poor communication is also likely to be part of the reason for strained relationships, limiting the improvement of patients and the quality of life of the carers.

These are all long-standing problems. Too often it seems to be assumed that if the carer has managed without breaking down in the first year, then the situation is under control; but the evidence from the carers' lives and anxieties contradicts this. In many respects the health and quality of life of the carers is worse when recovery slows down and stops. Apart from feeling physically exhausted, a third or more of the carers report that their health has deteriorated over the year following the stroke; they frequently suffer from sleeplessness, anxiety and mental strain. While these problems mount, resources for coping may diminish. For various reasons family and friends may call in less often, and do less than the carer feels they could do to help. There may be less money available, particularly if the patient or carer has had to change or give up employment;

this is one reason why a quarter or more of carers and their families suffer some financial loss after the stroke.

The effects of the stroke tend to be more deleterious to the health and lives of women carers than for men. This may be because men are fitter, or because they generally receive more outside help, especially with housework. Cultural expectations of women as carers are higher, which may be reflected in professionals being less likely to organize support for women, as well as by male carers being more inclined to accept help from others. Women living at home with their disabled husbands may be a particularly important group, amenable to counselling and organization of support by the primary health care team. The spouses of patients with communication impairments constitute another target group for general practitioners – they seem more likely to become socially isolated and poorly adjusted to the effects of the stroke.

IMPLICATIONS FOR GENERAL PRACTITIONERS

Much of the material presented in this chapter will come as no surprise to many doctors. General practitioners in the Greenwich health district were asked to identify the major longer-term problems for the carers of stroke patients. The four commonest problems that were mentioned were: emotional distress and frustration; burden and physical exhaustion of caring; restrictions on the carer's social life; and disruption of family roles and relationships. Many doctors identified problems in several aspects of life and clearly gave as much emphasis to psychosocial as to physical problems. Many of the responses indicated awareness of the breadth of the problems:

Other person will have to take on a lot: a big physical burden – may be reversal of domestic roles. Restriction on outings and holidays.

Continual stress – difficulty in getting relief except for holidays. Being inhibited about going out leads to their own social life being damaged and depression.

A restriction on physical activity for the whole family. Considerable emotional disturbance to patient and family. You're faced with a new person.

A major problem appears to be that this level of awareness may not be translated into contact with, and action for, the carers of stroke patients. Why do general practitioners and others in the primary health care team not appear to do more to prevent and alleviate problems faced by carers? A response that little can be done represents a profound misapprehension of both the opportunities available and the aspirations of carers, who do not expect miracles. What they do want is:

1. caring interest,
2. information about progress and skills for dealing with problems,
3. access to services and to financial benefits,
4. continuing support and understanding of their contribution.

General practitioners are 'continuing care' doctors and should be supported by an effective primary health care team. They have a professional interest in preventing longer-term problems. This should be based upon early contact with the carer to:

1. establish or redefine the relationship between doctor and carer;
2. identify the needs and preferences of carers (for information and services);
3. discuss current anxieties and realistic goals;
4. prepare the carer for common problems such as reorganizing domestic responsibilities, coping with changes in the patient's mood or behaviour;
5. provide reassurance that the doctor is interested and available.

Following this initial contact the general practitioner should return to assess circumstances, specifically when the patient is discharged from hospital, when formal rehabilitation ends, and about a year after the stroke when recovery has probably reached a plateau.

Many of the carers' problems will not be dealt with directly by the general practitioner because they require help from other people and services. However, as the carers' key contact the general practitioner should ensure that:

1. in most cases a social worker has seen the carer and is called in when circumstances change;
2. the help of district nurses, health visitors, bathing assistants and home helps is available, equally to men and women;
3. carers are informed about, and are helped to obtain, respite care;
4. carers know of, and can attend, support groups.

General practitioners should treat carers as important members of the primary care team. They need education and training, but above all they need *time* – to talk over problems, to make decisions, to learn new skills and to be free from their caring responsibilities. However, time is not usually the great healer; problems change in their priority, but seldom disappear. In adjusting to a stroke, carers may suffer many of the same handicaps as patients, and they could, equally, benefit from greater interest and help.

PRACTICAL POINTS

General practitioners should advise older patients and their families to let them know if any of them is admitted to hospital, and again to inform their doctor when the patient returns home. Carers often believe that the doctor knows this, but has simply not been in touch.

The general practitioner should visit the main carer at home not only to provide reassurance and 'caring interest', but also to identify needs and bring carers into contact with other services.

Members of the primary health care team can help carers to learn skills for rehabilitation and support of patients, and they can give information. All should be aware of local self-help groups to which carers may be referred and Chest, Heart and Stroke Association booklets should be made available to the carers.

A major aim in the management of stroke should be to prevent breakdown of the carer; a related aim must be to prevent breakdown in the relationship between patient and carer. The primary care team can help to put the patient's problems in some perspective, can advise on improving communication, and should help to organize opportunities for 'time-off' for the carers.

The expectations, priorities, resources and willingness of the carer change over time. Coming to terms with a stroke is a continuing process which therefore demands that the support of the general practitioner should express 'continuity of care'. Contact is particularly important in the first few weeks, after return from hospital, and at the end of the patient's period of physical recovery.

10

PRIMARY PREVENTION OF STROKE

The primary prevention of stroke is inextricably linked with the prevention of ischaemic heart disease and peripheral vascular disease. After age, hypertension is by far the most important single risk factor for stroke. General practitioners are ideally placed to use a 'high-risk' strategy; that is to identify and treat (usually with drugs) people who are at high risk of stroke. They can also provide the long-term management and follow-up such patients require. However, GPs are also able to apply the 'mass' stroke prevention strategy by reducing the level of risk factors (usually not with drugs, but by changes in lifestyle) in all the people registered with their practice. Getting people to stop smoking, lose weight, take more exercise and eat a healthier diet are areas where GPs – and their ancillary staff – should be very effective. With only relatively small changes in practice organization, it is possible to set up a simple but effective GP-based primary vascular disease prevention service.

This chapter is split into three sections: the aims and general principles of stroke prevention; the management of risk factors for stroke; and the various ways a practice can organize a simple but effective prevention programme.

STROKE PREVENTION – DEFINITIONS AND PRINCIPLES

Primary and secondary stroke prevention

Primary prevention is doing things which reduce the risk of stroke in people who haven't yet had one. Secondary prevention is preventing a second stroke in patients who have had a stroke in the past.

What are we trying to prevent and why?

It is very difficult to consider primary stroke prevention in isolation, because people at high risk of stroke are also at risk of ischaemic heart disease, peripheral vascular disease and death from a variety of vascular diseases (e.g. ruptured aortic aneurysm or 'sudden' presumed cardiovascular death). A successful GP-based primary prevention programme is likely to reduce morbidity and mortality not only from stroke, but also from other important vascular diseases.

Prevention is a rather abused term; in reality most of the measures discussed are likely to delay the onset of stroke rather than prevent it altogether. Furthermore, the aim should be to increase morbidity-free survival, and not merely to extend total lifespan.

'Mass' versus 'high-risk' strategy

There are two main ways of preventing disease. The 'mass' strategy attempts to reduce the level of a risk factor in the entire population by a small amount (Figure 10.1a) while the 'high risk' strategy attempts to identify and treat only the small number of individuals who have the highest levels of risk

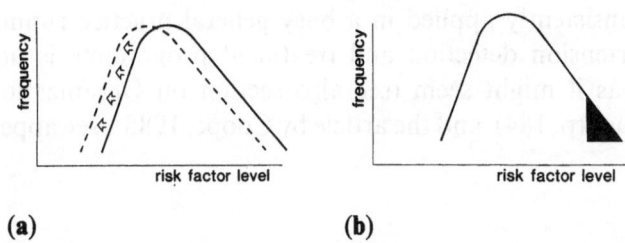

Figure 10.1 **(a)** The 'mass strategy' aims to lower the average level of the risk factor in the whole population by lowering the level in every individual by a small amount. **(b)** The 'high risk strategy' aims to identify the people at the highest levels of risk (shaded area) and give them specific drug treatments

(Figure 10.1b). The larger the number of people (and the healthier they are) that a particular measure is to be applied to, the safer it has to be, so that in general the 'mass strategy' has to rely on low-risk measures such as discouraging smoking, and reducing weight and cholesterol levels by diet. On the other hand, it is easier to justify the risks and expense of drugs (such as betablockers or aspirin) to prevent vascular events in the much smaller number of people at high risk. There are arguments in favour of both approaches which will be discussed further in relation to individual risk factors. The British GP is almost uniquely placed to adopt either approach in trying to prevent stroke, or indeed both, since they are certainly not mutually exclusive.

RISK FACTORS FOR TIA AND STROKE
(see also Chapter 1)

Hypertension

After age, hypertension is the single most important risk factor for stroke. It is particularly important because high blood pressure is very common in the general population. However, drawing up a sensible definition of hypertension which can be consistently applied in a busy general practice running a hypertension detection and treatment programme is not as easy as it might seem (see also section on Organization of practice (p. 184), and the article by Coope, 1985 – see appendix 4).

Problems defining hypertension

One way of defining hypertension is 'the level of blood pressure above which the risk of stroke is increased'. If one then defines a 'hypertensive' as someone with a blood pressure over 160/95 mmHg, then 'hypertensives' have approximately double the risk of stroke as 'normotensives'. However, this way of defining hypertension ignores the fact that the risk of stroke rises continuously with blood pressure, so that someone with a blood pressure of 150/90 is at higher risk of stroke (all other things being equal) than someone with a pressure of 120/80, even though both are 'normotensive'.

The majority of strokes are in fact attributable to the very large number of people with mild elevations of blood pressure rather than to the few with very high pressures (see Table 10.1). Rose has calculated that the life-saving benefits from a small reduction (2–3 mmHg) in the entire nation's average blood pressure would probably be equal to the benefits from antihypertensive drug treatment given to the relatively small number of people with 'hypertension'.

Thus the GP now has to consider not only the small number of patients on his list who have the sort of high blood pressure that requires drug treatment, but also the very large number with 'normal' or only slightly elevated pressures. Drug treatment in these last two groups certainly seems inappropriate, yet lowering their pressure might prevent a lot of vascular disease, particularly stroke (see section on treatment, p. 176).

Table 10.1 Population-attributable mortality from coronary heart disease and stroke arising at different levels of blood pressure

Diastolic BP	*Cumulative percentage of excess deaths attributable to hypertension*	
	---	---
(mmHg)	*Coronary heart disease*	*Stroke*
< 80	0	0
< 90	21	14
<100	47	25
<110	67	73
>110	100	100

Reproduced by kind permission of Professor G. Rose and the *British Medical Journal* (1981, **282**, 1847–1851)

Systolic or diastolic pressure?

Far too many doctors pay far too much attention to the diastolic blood pressure. The diastolic pressure is more difficult to measure accurately and repeatably than the systolic, and it is not as strong a predictor of stroke risk. Systolic hypertension with a 'normal' diastolic pressure (i.e. less than 95 mmHg), even in the elderly, is a risk factor for stroke.

How many readings?

Although data from the Framingham study have suggested that a single casual blood pressure reading is a reliable predictor of the *risk* of future blood pressure-related vascular events, few doctors would begin lifelong *treatment* of 'hypertension' on the basis of a single reading. The council of perfection (at least when deciding on whether drug treatment is needed or not) might suggest four or five readings over a few weeks before classing a patient as 'hypertensive' or not. A large proportion, perhaps one-third to one-half, of people with mild hypertension will revert over the next few years to having normal blood pressure levels without ever being treated.

Antihypertensive treatment – for whom, with what and by whom?

Another way to define 'hypertension' is the level of blood pressure above which treatment does more good than harm. That level will be determined by a variety of factors such as the age of the patient, the presence of other risk factors, and the balance between the 'costs' (side-effects from the treatment) and the 'benefits' (reduced morbidity and mortality).

However, let there be no doubt about the potential value of treating even mild hypertension. Three recent trials have shown that antihypertensive drug treatment reduces the risk of stroke in patients with mild to moderate hypertension by about half. However, although the relative reduction in stroke risk sounds impressive, it is the absolute reduction which is the more important. In the relatively young and healthy patients studied in the MRC mild-to-moderate hypertension trial, the difference in the stroke rates between the treated and placebo groups was 1.6 per 1000 patient-years, but in the older, higher-risk patients of the European Working Party on Hypertension in the Elderly (EWPHE) study the difference was 26 per 1000 patient-years.

These results suggest that drug treatment, in younger patients with mild hypertension who are free of other risk factors, does not confer worthwhile benefit, though blood pressure reduction by other means, such as reduction of weight and alcohol intake, might be fruitful, largely because they are safer and cheaper. Reducing either the salt or saturated fat content of the diet, increasing physical fitness, and relaxation exercises have all been suggested as further measures that could be used, though all require more detailed study.

On the other hand, in patients in whom the absolute risk of stroke is higher (such as patients aged over 60) drug treatment becomes much more worthwhile. Thus in the MRC trial and the EWHPE trials 850 and 90 patient-years of treatment respectively were needed to prevent one stroke. In other words, the benefits of treating hypertension are greatest in a high-risk group such as the elderly.

Unfortunately, although the benefits are potentially greater in the elderly, so too are the side-effects. The published trials in hypertensives have suggested that both diuretics and beta-blockers carry a fairly high risk of side-effects, and that beta-blockers have not yet been shown to have the favourable effect on cardiac mortality which had been predicted.

In deciding on how to deal with hypertension in the practice as a whole, one needs to be able to split the patients into three groups: the definitely hypertensive who need drug treatment; the borderline patients whose pressure is not high enough to warrant drug therapy, but who might benefit from management of other risk factors; and the people with definitely normal blood pressure. The first group needs close supervision, the second perhaps an annual review, and the normotensives a check-up every 5 years. This is the 'three box' system devised by Dr John Coope (see Table 10.2 and Figure 10.2).

Finally, many of the clinical trials have used carefully trained nurses to screen, treat and follow up the patients. Nurses have proved themselves efficient, thorough and consistent in the long-term management of patients with hypertension. There is much to be said for a nurse-run hypertension clinic based in the practice (see Chapter 11).

Heart disease

People with cardiac abnormalities are at greater risk of stroke than those without. Hypertensive heart disease (left ventricular hypertrophy on an ECG, for example) is associated with an increased risk of both cerebral infarction and cerebral haemorrhage. Lesions which can release emboli into the arterial circulation, such as mural thrombus on a recent myocardial

Table 10.2 The 'three box' system

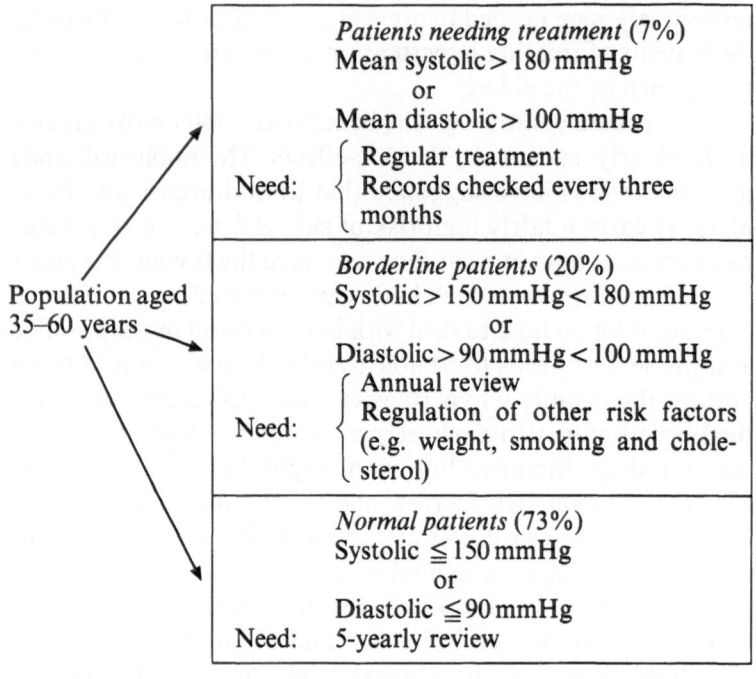

Patients needing treatment (7%)
Mean systolic > 180 mmHg
or
Mean diastolic > 100 mmHg

Need:
{
Regular treatment
Records checked every three
months
}

Borderline patients (20%)
Systolic > 150 mmHg < 180 mmHg
or
Diastolic > 90 mmHg < 100 mmHg

Need:
{
Annual review
Regulation of other risk factors
(e.g. weight, smoking and cholesterol)
}

Normal patients (73%)
Systolic ≤ 150 mmHg
or
Diastolic ≤ 90 mmHg

Need: 5-yearly review

Population aged
35–60 years

NB: the criteria for allocation to the boxes may vary from time to
time depending on the evidence in the literature, or from practice to
practice depending on the consensus of the team.

infarction or thrombus in a fibrillating left atrium, increase
the risk of cerebral infarction. However, in a patient with a
cardiac lesion and a stroke, one cannot necessarily assume
either that the stroke was due to cerebral infarction or that,
even if the stroke was due to cerebral infarction, the infarction
was due to embolism from the heart to the brain. The cardiac
lesions associated with embolism to the brain are discussed in
Chapter 2. (See also Chapter 5.)

The treatment of cardiac lesions to prevent stroke is a
difficult topic to summarize briefly. A few points can be made
clearly:

HYPERTENSION

SURNAME	FORENAMES	DATE OF BIRTH

ADDRESS

SUMMARY OF HISTORY

....

....

....

....

....

....

FAMILY HISTORY

....

SMOKING HISTORY

....

....

ANTIDEPRESSIVE	STEROIDS	CONTRACEPTIVE

BASIC DATA   DATE

B.P.	F.B.C.	CHOLESTEROL	
WEIGHT	Na.	LIPOPROTEINS	
FUNDI	K.	URINE	Alb.
			Sugar
HEART FAILURE	UREA	E.C.G.	
ABDOMINAL BRUIT	CREATININE	CHEST FILM	
FEMORAL PULSES	BL. SUGAR	I.V.P.	

Figure 10.2 Hypertension card – used in the 'three box' system (Courtesy of Dr John Coope)

1. There is some evidence that treating patients with aspirin
   1 g daily in the months and years after a myocardial infarction may reduce the risk of stroke by about 25%. Further
   evidence is required, particularly on whether smaller doses
   with a lower risk of dose-related gastrointestinal side-effects
   are equally effective.
2. Patients with any of the following cardiac lesions should
   probably be given long-term oral anticoagulant therapy:
   atrial fibrillation plus rheumatic heart disease,
   artificial heart valve prosthesis,
   recent myocardial infarction followed by TIA or cerebral
   infarction (treat for a few months only).
3. There is no convincing evidence either for or against the
   use of anticoagulants in patients with:
   atrial fibrillation not associated with rheumatic valvular
   disease,
   mitral incompetence, mitral leaflet prolapse without AF,
   aortic valve disease.
4. Anticoagulants should not be used in patients with subacute
   bacterial endocarditis.

Peripheral vascular disease

It is no surprise that the presence of symptomatic atheromatous arterial disease in the legs (e.g. intermittent claudication) signals an increased risk of atheromatous disease
elsewhere (e.g. in the cerebral blood supply). Patients with
intermittent claudication can be identified easily, without
complicated tests, and are a useful group to study since they
have a high absolute risk of cardiovascular and cerebrovascular events. However, no simple widely applicable
treatment given to these patients has yet been shown to reduce
the risk of stroke or myocardial infarction. Aspirin and beta-
blockers appear the most promising treatments, and some
studies are in progress, although beta-blockers may make
circulatory problems in the legs worse. Since the value of

treatment is uncertain, it is open to debate whether one should or should not screen for people with this particular risk factor.

TIA as a risk factor for stroke

TIA are a potent risk factor for strokes; people with TIA, have a risk of stroke roughly five times that of people without. However, TIA are a symptom of cerebrovascular disease, so treating people who have had TIA is not, strictly speaking, primary prevention of cerebrovascular disease. On the other hand, TIA are a risk factor for both stroke *and* cardiovascular disease, can be fairly easily identified (Chapter 3) and treatment is straightforward (Chapter 5). One could make out a case for making a systematic search for patients in the practice who have had TIA at some time in the past.

Asymptomatic carotid bruit

People with an asymptomatic carotid arterial bruit are at increased risk of stroke. However, there can often be a significant atheromatous lesion in the internal carotid artery which is capable of causing a stroke by embolization or occlusion, yet does not cause a bruit (see Chapter 2). Furthermore, a bruit does not necessarily imply the presence of a significant atheromatous lesion.

If a patient has a carotid bruit but has not had a stroke or TIA, then the absolute risk of stroke is low, and the risk of a stroke from cerebral angiography (and carotid endarterectomy if a 'significant' lesion is found) is much greater. These patients should therefore *not* be operated on. We do not know whether using drugs (such as aspirin or beta-blockers) gives a worthwhile reduction in the risk of subsequent stroke and cardiovascular death, although presumably the modification of other risk factors (e.g. hypertension) does.

Smoking

Cigarette smoking (and probably pipe and cigar smoking too) is a potent risk factor for ischaemic heart disease and peripheral vascular disease. Its relation to TIA and stroke is less certain. Encouraging people to stop smoking will prevent a lot of heart attacks and probably some strokes. The burden of smoking-related diseases is so high that anti-smoking advice should come high on the GP's list of prevention priorities. Having said that, the government could make a very substantial contribution to the 'mass strategy' by increasing the cost of tobacco, by forbidding tobacco use in public places (and in hospitals and civil service offices), and by banning tobacco advertising and sponsorship.

Cholesterol and lipids

Elevated blood cholesterol is a risk factor for ischaemic heart disease. The relationship between blood fats and cerebrovascular disease is much less clear. However, compelling evidence is emerging that a 10% lowering of blood cholesterol level by either diet or drugs may reduce vascular mortality and morbidity by around 10–20%.

Should GPs merely encourage everyone on the practice list to reduce their intake of saturated fat, or should they screen or case-find for hypercholesterolaemia? If one was going to screen, a first step might be to screen all males over 40 for hypercholesterolaemia, and treat people with raised levels by diet and careful blood level monitoring, going on to lipid-lowering drugs if diet alone failed.

In our opinion, every GP surgery should at least provide information to all those who attend the surgery on the value of a low-saturated fat/high-fibre diet. Posters in the waiting room, and leaflets which patients can take away, cost little or nothing. More enthusiastic practices might use case-finding for hypercholesterolaemics, referring those picked up to a dietitian. Screening the whole practice for hyper-cholesterolaemia should probably take a lower priority for the moment. Opportunistic health promotion concerning diet and lifestyle should probably be part of any consultation (in hospital or general practice) when time permits.

Indeed, it appears that the GP is the most effective and respected motivator for lifestyle modification, and it would therefore be logical to reduce the list size of doctors demonstrably practising preventive medicine.

Diabetes

Although diabetics have approximately twice the risk of stroke of non-diabetics, there is no really hard evidence that improved control of hyperglycaemia reduces that risk. On the other hand, audit of the quality of diabetic management in the practice, or systematic early detection of asymptomatic diabetics by case-finding, are both worth considering as part of a vascular disease prevention effort.

The oral contraceptive pill

The proportion of strokes which can be attributed to the effects of the 'pill' is extremely small. Nonetheless, inappropriate pill use in high-risk women is an avoidable cause of stroke. It would seem reasonable, provided the extra work does not get in the way of other practice prevention efforts, to make periodic systematic checks that women are advised to come off the pill when they pass the age of 35, if they are smokers, or if they are at risk of stroke for some other reason. Much of this sort of work can be delegated by the GP to a prevention nurse (see section on practice organization, p. 184).

Elevated haematocrit

Both polycythaemia rubra vera (PRV), and rather more modest elevations of the haematocrit ($>50\%$) not due to PRV, are a risk factor for TIA and cerebral infarction. PRV requires immunosuppressive treatment and venesection. As we do not know whether venesecting people with a high 'normal' haematocrit (45–50%) provides a worthwhile reduction in the risk of stroke, there is no need to screen for this risk factor.

Other risk factors

Various dietary factors such as the intake of salt, minerals, vitamins (especially vitamin C) and alcohol have been related to stroke in various ways. Unfortunately the fraction of all strokes attributable to each factor, separately or in aggregate, is unknown; it is probably small. So their manipulation, with the possible exceptions of alcohol and vitamin C, is not a priority at present. A reduction in the nation's intake of alcohol would be desirable, but the most effective way of achieving this would be through government-initiated measures, rather than through GP-based intervention. Increased tax on alcohol, reduced availability through retail sales outlets, and a ban on advertising could all be applied by a government committed to improving the health of the nation.

SETTING UP A STROKE PREVENTION PROGRAMME IN THE PRACTICE

Getting started

Every general practice is different, with its own strengths and weaknesses. A stroke prevention programme will inevitably bring changes in practice organization. However small the changes may be, the programme must be tailored to fit into a particular practice and to capitalize on its strengths. Everyone in the practice team has to be convinced of the value of the programme for it to be successful, so a lot of work has to go into explaining the background and finding simple workable solutions to the practical problems. Solutions to the same problem will vary from practice to practice, so we can only offer general guidelines and the assurance that 'it can be done'. The Oxfordshire Area Health Authority has pioneered a system to help practices through the difficult initial stages of setting up a prevention programme. A 'facilitator' visits the practice and can provide the help outlined in Table 10.3. Anyone interested in this idea should write to Elaine Fullard, Oxfordshire Prevention of Heart Attack and Stroke Project, Community Health Offices, Radcliffe Infirmary, Woodstock Road, Oxford OX2 6HE.

Table 10.3

Science
Provide practical definitions of hypertension, obesity, other risk factors.
Help select the risk factors worth looking for
Up-to-date advice on current treatment of high risk groups

Organization
Arrange informal contact with other practices who have already started
Suggest organizational method to suit a particular practice
Provide sample risk factor cards to put in records (Figure 10.3)
Help organize practice audit of risk factor management
Provide sample information leaflets to give to the patients on diet, smoking (and ways to give up) etc.
Advise on ways to cover extra staff costs
Ways of screening/case-finding

Enthusiam
Show that it can be done!

It can be done

Many doctors are convinced of the need to start on preventive work, but either can't quite summon up the energy to get started or don't really know where to begin. The story below is fictional, but illustrates the problems!

HEALTH SUMMARY   **MALE**

Name

D.O.B.		SMWD		No.	

Own Occupation
Partner's Occupation

Date	Date	Date	
1st B/P	2nd B/P	3rd B/P	Mean if applicable

Weight	Ideal Weight	Height

Smoker	Cigarettes	Pipe	Since 19
Non Smoker	Never	Stopped 19	

Family History of CVA or MI

Diabetes	Yes	Insulin	OHD	Diet
	No			

Date of Tetanus	1st	2nd	3rd	Booster

Urine Date	Protein	Sugar

Alcohol

Allergies

Notes / Past Operations

Figure 10.3 Risk factor card used by the Oxfordshire Prevention of Heart Attack and Stroke Project (courtesy of Elaine Fullard)

Dr Keen joins a four-man practice in a small market town as the junior partner. He has just finished his trainee year and wants to start a stroke prevention programme. All the partners agree that this seems like a good idea, but the senior partner is quite reasonably worried about the cost and extra workload. The other two partners aren't sure how many risk factors to screen for. Dr Keen feels he is up against a brick wall. Fortunately, he meets Dr Smart from the rival practice which has just taken on an extra practice nurse to run a hypertension screening and treatment clinic. Dr Smart suggests contact with the Oxford Project. The facilitator from Oxford visits the practice. She agrees with the senior partner that space is a bit of a problem, but is able to suggest various ways to minimize the cost of the extra staff. She provides background data on risk factors and some definitions used by other practices that seem to work well. The facilitator talks to the practice ancillary staff to explain the problems they are likely to face and arranges for them to visit a practice where a prevention programme is already running. The whole practice decides to give it a go, but with a fairly simple scheme that does not require extra staff. A year later, enthusiasm for the programme from the patients and practice staff encourages them to take on a 'prevention' nurse. The senior partner organizes the nurse's work so that her net cost to the practice is nil.

The basics of getting the practice organized for prevention

(a) *Good records.* An individual patient summary card, which includes information on risk factors, is a good start. If available on the front of the notes, it can serve as a reminder to the GP to check on any risk factors which have not been checked in previous surgery visits. Thus a consultation about a sprained ankle (if the surgery is not too busy) may provide the opportunity to check the patient's blood pressure and smoking history. This sort of system is best maintained by a well-trained 'records nurse' or clerk, who is given time each week for 'servicing' the notes, systematically ensuring that patients' notes have risk factor cards correctly filled in, and possibly even leaving reminders for the doctor about items to be checked at future visits.

(b) *Age–sex register*. An age–sex register (ASR) is a very useful tool in any screening programme because it allows at-risk people to be identified and then invited to attend for screening (e.g. women over 35 for cervical smears, men over 40 for hypertension screening, etc.). However, ASRs do require regular maintenance, and the practice manager or secretary should be fully aware that a carefully kept up-to-date ASR maximizes the practice's standard of care and income.

(c) *'Opportunistic' case-finding.* This trendy phrase, popular with GP trainers and course organizers, merely describes the easiest way of picking up people at risk of stroke. Between 70 and 90% of all people registered with a practice are likely to attend the surgery within the space of a year or so. Such visits offer the opportunity to check blood pressure, smoking habits and weight. A summary card with spaces for the relevant risk factors may encourage enthusiasts to make sure that risk factors have been checked recently. Opportunistic case-finding is a relatively painless and effective way of picking up pre-viously undetected hypertensives during routine consultations. Data from the Oxfordshire Community Stroke Project suggest that a large proportion of patients with two other important risk factors, TIA and atrial fibrillation, could also be picked up by this method.

(d) *Screening*. Screening, used in this context, implies a more active search for those at risk. The extra effort need not be great. The easiest method is to check the records of patients likely to be at risk (say those aged over 40) preferably using the ASR, and invite those who have not had risk factors measured recently to attend for examination. This sort of request is often greeted enthusiastically by people ('it shows my doctor cares for me'). A more vigorous programme might involve inviting all the over-40s to attend for screening, not just those who haven't recently been to the surgery.

(e) *Screening or case-finding for patients with TIA?* It is diffi-cult to advise on the best way of finding patients in the practice who have had TIA. Case-finding may miss quite a few, since a significant proportion of patients with TIA probably do not seek medical attention, or forget about attacks months or years previously. On the other hand, screening the healthy population is notoriously difficult and laborious, because a lot of elderly patients with non-specific 'funny turns' will report symptoms that might be TIA and generate a lot of false-positives. On balance, case-finding seems the best approach at present.

The role of ancillary staff

Getting the whole team involved. If the practice has an active prevention programme, the ancillary staff may wish to be involved, and may well get extra job satisfaction. Their participation will reduce the workload for the doctor. For example, the practice nurse could set aside 2 hours a week for a 'health check' clinic for checking risk factors. The practice receptionist could invite patients as they arrive at the surgery (especially those who have not had a risk factor card filled out) to attend at a later date for a 'health check' with the nurse. Every few months the nurse (or practice manager) might then, using the ASR, identify people who have not attended the surgery and send them an appointment to see the practice nurse.

Taking on extra staff. So far, all the prevention work discussed can be done by the existing practice staff. However, in practices which do not have their full complement of staff it may cost very little extra to take on a 'prevention nurse'; the Family Practitioner Committee will reimburse 70% of her salary, and 40% of the rest is tax-deductible. In addition, fees for cervical smears and tetanus immunizations are likely to make up the balance of her salary. The prevention nurse can than take on the organization and running of the work in the practice. Dr John Coope describes a simple and extremely effective 'three box' system for the detection and management of hypertension which is almost entirely run by the prevention nurse in his practice (see Table 10.2, on p. 178).

How much effort should be put into prevention?

It is better to start with a relatively modest prevention programme and make a success of it than to begin ambitiously and fail. Success may encourage the practice staff to try a more extensive programme once they see how much patients appreciate practice-based prevention work. Table 10.4 gives suggestions for changes matched to the practice's level of enthusiasm.

Table 10.4

The basics
Measure BP at every opportunity
Encourage smokers to stop
Weigh patients
Have posters and leaflets on healthy diet in the waiting room
Keep an eye out for patients with TIA

More advanced
Set up an age–sex register
Summary sheet of past illnesses for each patient record
Risk factor card on every patient over 40 (Figure 10.3)
Get receptionist to invite people over 40 to attend for a health check
    by the nurse, when they come to surgery
Get a dietitian to arrange 'healthy diet' meetings

For the enthusiasts
Take on a 'prevention nurse'
Audit the state of the risk factor cards
Invite people with blank cards to attend for a health check
'Three box' system for hypertension

For the future?
Screen for hypercholesterolaemia
Run lifestyle management classes in the practice

PRACTICAL POINTS

Hypertension is by far the most important risk factor for stroke; most of one's energy should be aimed at its prevention, detection and treatment.

In people with borderline blood pressure, drug therapy is probably inappropriate but management of other risk factors is very important.

The value of detecting and treating people with other risk factors is less clear; individual practices may wish to look for people with heart disease, peripheral vascular disease or hypercholesterolaemia.

A variety of methods can be used to detect patients at high risk; most do not require much extra work.

GPs should think about encouraging everyone on the practice list to stop smoking, improve their diet, achieve an ideal weight and lead a healthier lifestyle as part of the effort towards the mass prevention of vascular disease.

Good practice records, summary cards and an age–sex register make prevention work much easier.

Extra staff to help with prevention may cost the practice very little, or nothing.

11

SECONDARY PREVENTION OF STROKE

Secondary prevention after stroke requires a different approach from primary prevention for several reasons: the numbers involved are much smaller; it may be difficult for the GP to select appropriate treatment; systematic follow-up is important and must be organized efficiently.

SECONDARY STROKE PREVENTION – A DIFFERENT SET OF PROBLEMS

Secondary prevention for the few vs. primary prevention for the many?

The first problem for the GP is deciding on priorities – is it best to channel limited resources into primary prevention for the many or secondary prevention for the few? In a practice list of 2000 patients with a typical age distribution, there would be:

Number of new strokes/TIA each year   = 5
Number of stroke/TIA survivors on the practice
list on a given day   = 15–20
Number of patients in the practice with
hypertension requiring treatment.   = 40–50
Number of patients at risk of stroke   = 50–200
Number of people in the practice who might
potentially benefit from screening for hypertension,
say all those aged 35–65   = 650

What are we trying to prevent in whom?

Prevention of heart disease after stroke. Most people who survive from a first stroke eventually die, not from a recurrent stroke, but from myocardial infarction and other *cardio*vascular events (e.g. cardiac failure). The aim of secondary prevention must therefore be to reduce mortality and morbidity from all forms of vascular disease, and not just from stroke.

When is it NOT worth trying to prevent another stroke? When a patient presents with a stroke or TIA, the first thing to decide is 'is it worth preventing recurrent vascular events in this patient?' Patients who were already severely disabled before their first stroke (e.g. because of arthritis), or who have had a major disabling stroke, be it due to infarction or haemorrhage, may have little to lose from a further stroke, so preventive efforts for them should perhaps be less than vigorous. Nonetheless, the practice organization should somehow ensure that the decision to be inactive is kept under review and is reversed if unexpected recovery occurs (see section on Practice organization). A uniform follow-up system applied to all patients with stroke, irrespective of the severity, may help overcome the problem.

SPECIFIC TREATMENTS FOR SPECIFIC TYPES OF STROKE OR TIA

Simple clinical selection criteria

If the patient is not severely disabled, then the next question is 'what preventive treatment does this patient need?' Apart from the control of hypertension, preventive measures after stroke depend on the pathological type of stroke – the treatments for cerebral infarction and primary intracerebral haemorrhage (PICH) are, not surprisingly, different. Unfortunately CT scanning is not widely available, so GPs and most hospital doctors seldom know the pathological type of stroke when trying to decide on treatment. If the patient fits into one of the following five groups, then referral to hospital for specialist assessment, CT scanning and angiography may be indicated.

1. Carotid surgery

If the event was a TIA or minor stroke, then carotid surgery is a possibility, so it may be worth referring patients for further assessment (see Chapter 5), provided they are generally fit and able to withstand surgery.

2. Cardiac lesions

If there is a significant cardiac lesion (Chapter 2), referral for a full cardiac assessment is important, followed by CT within 2 or 3 weeks of onset to exclude primary intracerebral haemorrhage, particularly if anticoagulants are considered necessary.

3. Patients already on/needing to start anticoagulants

Patients already on anticoagulants sometimes suffer strokes. Further management of the anticoagulants is not possible until one knows whether the stroke was due to infarction, in which case it is reasonable to continue, or haemorrhage, in which case they should be stopped. Deep venous thrombosis and pulmonary embolism are common complications of stroke, and again CT scanning, to exclude intracranial haemorrhage, is mandatory before anticoagulants are started.

4. Does one need to do a CT scan before starting aspirin?

Although occasional patients with 'TIA' lasting less than 24 hours have been found to have very small intracerebral haemorrhages, these are so rare that it is quite reasonable to start patients with clear-cut TIA on aspirin. However, we do not know whether starting a patient with a haemorrhagic stroke on aspirin is likely to increase the intracranial bleeding or not; trials in progress may help. In other words, we do not know whether it is reasonable to give aspirin to a patient who has had a stroke, but not a CT scan; *probably* it is not a good idea.

Is there an alternative to CT scanning? The Allen Score (Chapter 4), which uses simple clinical data, does improve the chances of getting the pathological type of stroke correct. Unfortunately, it is still not reliable enough at excluding primary intracerebral haemorrhage for it to be useful in patients who require oral anticoagulants. It *may* be possible to use it to exclude primary intracerebral haemorrhage in patients who are suitable for aspirin therapy, but the score's reliability now needs to be tested in a large clinical trial.

5. Suspected haemorrhagic stroke

If the patient is hypertensive, and the CT scan shows the typical appearance of a hypertensive bleed, then no further investigation is necessary. Assessment of clotting factors and cerebral angiography may be necessary in non-hypertensive intracerebral haemorrhage. Careful monitoring of blood pressure is important in all cases.

Subarachnoid haemorrhage is uncommon (Chapter 1) and the 50% or so of patients who survive the initial bleed (Chapter 6) will generally require admission to hospital and, if fit enough, transfer to a neurological or neurosurgical unit for angiography and surgery.

ORGANIZING SECONDARY STROKE PREVENTION IN THE PRACTICE

The practical problems

This and the next section illustrate how much successful secondary prevention relies on accurate diagnosis and well-organized follow-up.

> Mr Timber, a 66-year-old retired carpenter, woke one morning and found that he had difficulty finding words, and weakness of the right hand. He smoked 20 cigarettes a day. His blood pressure was 180/105. The heart was normal. The GP sent off blood for full blood count, ESR, glucose, syphilis serology, and organized a chest X-ray and ECG. The GP explained the diagnosis and asked the patient to return. On his return a week later, Mr Timber reported that his speech and hand had recovered completely. His blood pressure was 170/100 (i.e. likely to need long-term treatment for hypertension, though it might be worth rechecking once more before starting treatment). Since he had made such a good recovery, the GP felt it would be worth referring him to the local neurologist. The neurologist agreed that it was a stroke and the CT scan showed a small cerebral infarct. Cerebral angiography showed an ulcerated atheromatous plaque at the origin of the left internal carotid artery. The patient was entered in the European carotid surgery trial and drew 'no-surgery'. The neurologist recommended aspirin 300 mg daily, and referred the patient back to the GP for control of his risk factors. The GP persuaded Mr Timber to give up smoking and controlled his hypertension with a diuretic. Mr Timber remained well for the next 6 years and then died suddenly from a presumed myocardial infarct.

This utopian fable illustrates how things should go in an ideal world. The GP provided successful long-term follow-up of the risk factors, and the patient had a long spell free of symptoms before his death at the age of 72. The next case shows a (true) example of how even the best may fail:

> A 40-year-old factory worker suddenly became very dizzy and unsteady. He requested a home visit. The GP examined him, diagnosed 'labyrinthitis' and treated him with vestibular sedatives. Because the symptoms cleared up over a few days the patient did not go back to the GP for a follow-up visit. A few months later the patient was admitted to hospital with a moderately severe brainstem stroke. His blood pressure on admission was 220/140 and the fundi showed some small haemorrhages. His hypertension was treated with a beta-blocker. Angiography was not performed because the event was not in the carotid territory.

This case illustrates how easy it can be to miss an opportunity to prevent a disabling stroke. In retrospect it is easy to see that the first episode of dizziness and unsteadiness was probably a mild brainstem stroke. Although the GP did not check the blood pressure at the first visit there might have been an opportunity to do so at a follow-up visit. Unfortunately, as the patient's symptoms had resolved, he quite reasonably did not bother to go back to his GP for a follow-up appointment. It is possible that if the hypertension had been detected at the first visit, or at a follow-up, the second stroke could have been avoided, or at least delayed.

A careful risk factor assessment for every patient

We do not know as much as we would like to about the factors which predict recurrence of stroke. However, it is reasonable to assume that the presence of any of the risk factors discussed in Chapter 10 is likely to increase the risk of serious vascular events. The difficulty is knowing by how much the risk is increased, and whether the increase is big enough to warrant the hazard of side-effects that any treatment might cause (e.g. stroke from carotid endarterectomy, intracerebral haem-

Table 11.1   Risk factor management after stroke

Definitely worth doing in all cases
Treat moderate to severe hypertension
Advise against cigarette smoking
Advise on weight control and healthy diet (high fibre, saturated fat
    30% of calories)

Patients with CT-confirmed cerebral infarction
Consider carotid endarterectomy if stroke is mild (see Chapter 5)
Anticoagulants for patients with atrial fibrillation and rheumatic
    heart disease or recent MI or valve prosthesis.
Give aspirin 300 mg daily

Patients with CT-proven intracranial haemorrhage
Monitor blood pressure and treat accordingly

Don't
Anticoagulate if atrial fibrillation and no other heart disease,
    especially if contraindications present (e.g. not possible to exclude
    intracranial haemorrhage by CT, age > 75, hypertension, peptic
    ulcer, confusion, or no reasonable prothrombin-measuring service
    available at local hospital)
Harass elderly patients about having to stop pipe/cigars
Give cerebral 'vasoactive' drugs (cyclospasmol, hydergine, trental)
Give dipyridamole (Persantin) or sulphinpyrazone (Anturan)

---

orrhage from anticoagulants or aspirin). Table 11.1 sum-
marizes some suggested do's and don't's in risk factor management after stroke.

Improving the organization of post-stroke and TIA care

In one way, secondary stroke prevention is easier to cope with
than primary stroke prevention because the patients almost
always (but not invariably) seek medical attention after their
stroke or TIA, so there are no worries about having to screen
for undetected disease. Furthermore, someone who has just
had a stroke is likely to be more motivated than an asymptomatic person to do something about his or her health. On the

other hand, keeping track of such patients, and making sure that risk factors are followed up consistently in each and every one of them after the acute phase is over, is more difficult. Although many practices have age–sex registers to help with primary prevention and screening, far fewer have disease registers which are so important for secondary prevention.

Suggestions for improving secondary prevention in the practice

(a) *Consider the diagnosis more often.* A greater awareness of the wide variety of clinical presentations of stroke and especially TIA (Chapters 3 and 4) is a very important first step. If the practice agrees to set up a stroke prevention programme, awareness in all the team members does tend to rise, at least at first, though it may be difficult to keep up the enthusiasm.

(b) *A basic risk factor assessment for every patient.* Assessment of risk factors by clinical assessment and a few basic investigations (see Chapter 3) are worthwhile in all but the moribund.

(c) *Follow-up.* Many patients who make a good recovery after their first stroke may not call the GP out after the first consultation. These are the very patients who have most to lose from a recurrent stroke, and in whom secondary prevention is most likely to be particularly worthwhile. A system of follow-up to ensure that risk factors are being successfully dealt with after 1 month, 6 months, 1 year and annually thereafter is worth considering. The assessment should be made simple enough for a nurse or health visitor to do.

(d) *Disease register – audit of management.* A disease register need not be complicated (see Table 11.2). The vascular register should ideally be the responsibility of a prevention nurse, who would keep reminding the staff of the need to look out for new cases, would monitor correspondence from hospitals, would keep the register up to date and would ensure completeness of

Table 11.2 Disease register

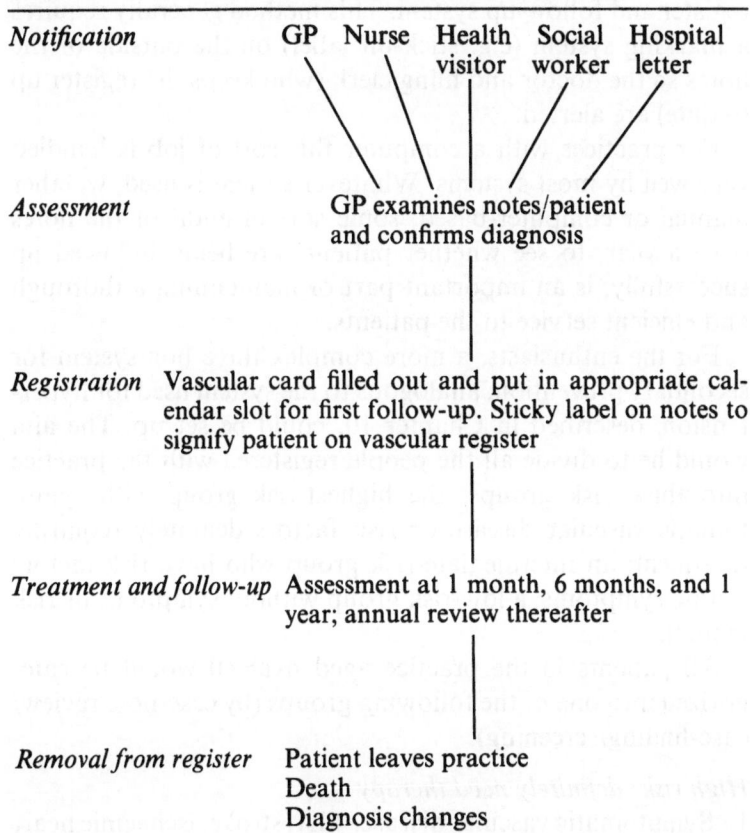

Notification	GP	Nurse	Health visitor	Social worker	Hospital letter

Assessment	GP examines notes/patient and confirms diagnosis

Registration	Vascular card filled out and put in appropriate calendar slot for first follow-up. Sticky label on notes to signify patient on vascular register

Treatment and follow-up	Assessment at 1 month, 6 months, and 1 year; annual review thereafter

Removal from register	Patient leaves practice
	Death
	Diagnosis changes

follow-up. A receptionist or 'prevention nurse' (Chapter 10) could make out a card for each new stroke or TIA patient at the time of presentation. A box could be divided into 12 sections, one for each month, so that the card of a patient who has a stroke in June would be filed in the July slot and an appointment made for the 1-month follow-up in July. After the follow-up appointment the card could be moved 6 months on into the January slot. At the end of July the slot would be checked to make sure that all that month's follow-ups had been done. The box would therefore provide a simple disease register and follow-up system. This method generally requires a marking system (e.g. stick-on label) on the outside of the notes so the doctor and filing clerk (who keeps the register up to date) are alerted.

For practices with a computer this sort of job is handled very well by most systems. Whatever system is used, whether manual or computer-based, some sort of audit of the notes once a year, to see whether patients are being followed up successfully, is an important part of maintaining a thorough and efficient service to the patients.

For the enthusiasts, a more complex three box system for secondary prevention, analogous to the system used for hypertension, described in Chapter 10, could be set up. The aim would be to divide all the people registered with the practice into three risk groups: the highest-risk group with symptomatic vascular disease or risk factors definitely requiring treatment: an intermediate-risk group who have risk factors but no symptoms: a low-risk group without symptoms or risk factors.

All patients in the practice aged over 40 would be categorized into one of the following groups (by case-note review/ case-finding/screening).

High risk: definitely need therapy
1. Symptomatic vascular disease: TIA, stroke, ischaemic heart disease, atrial fibrillation with rheumatic heart disease, intermittent claudication
   or
2. Risk factors requiring treatment; e.g. moderate to severe hypertension (systolic > 180 mmHg and/or diastolic > 100 mmHg), diabetes mellitus
ACTION: regular treatment and follow-up

Modest risk: need advice and careful risk factor follow-up
1. Asymptomatic vascular disease: 'silent' MI on ECG, non-rheumatic atrial fibrillation, asymptomatic carotid/femoral bruit or absent foot pulses

or

2. Risk factors not necessarily requiring drug treatment: mild hypertension, smoking, hypercholesterolaemia

ACTION: Careful advice on diet, ideal weight, smoking and exercise, with annual follow-up

Low risk:

1. None of the above

ACTION: Five- or 10-year review.

The definition of each of the risk groups will vary from time to time with the evidence available in the literature and the consensus of the team.

PRACTICAL POINTS

Secondary prevention is concerned with preventing *cardio*vascular events as well as strokes.

Every stroke patient deserves a basic assessment of risk factors, particularly if the stroke is mild and there is much to lose from a recurrent stroke.

Early and accurate diagnosis of mild stroke and TIA is very important. Careful follow-up with attention to risk factors is also vital.

Stroke patients should not be given anticoagulants or perhaps even aspirin, until a CT scan (within 2 or 3 weeks of the onset) has ruled out an intracerebral haemorrhage.

Ideally the primary care team should organize a systematic follow-up system for all stroke and TIA patients.

A simple disease register can be very useful.

APPENDIX 1

GLOSSARY OF TERMS WHICH ARE SOMETIMES MIS-USED OR MISUNDERSTOOD

Absolute risk (see risk).

Activities of daily living are everyday activities such as washing, dressing and going to the toilet. Various scales to measure these 'ADL' are available and we used the Barthel system (see appendix 2).

Adjustment reaction is a state of emotional arousal characterized by anxiety, distress and tension. Usually closely related in time to the provoking stress, transient and self-limiting.

Age-adjusted incidence (see incidence).

Age-specific incidence (see incidence).

Age-standardized incidence (see incidence).

Agraphia is the inability to write not because of weakness, clumsiness, or sensory loss in the hand but because there is a problem with language such that spelling is impaired and words cannot be expressed on the page.

Alexia (or dyslexia) is the inability to read because words do not make sense, rather than because they cannot be seen properly.

Amaurosis fugax is the *symptom* of transient monocular visual loss which may be due to ischaemia, or various ocular pathologies. If due to ischaemia it is one type of transient ischaemic attack.

Aphasia (see dysphasia) is inability or difficulty in speaking because of a language problem and not because of articulatory difficulty. Incorrect words may be used, words may come out in the wrong order, nonsense words are used, or the patient may not be able to think of words to express himself.

Apraxia is inability to do something (such as dressing, or using a pen) because there is a problem with putting together a learned movement; power, co-ordination, and sensation are normal.

Arteriovenous malformation (AVM) is an abnormal collection of blood vessels and may be a few millimetres to a few centimetres in diameter.

Attributable risk (see risk).

Cardiovascular disease is any disorder affecting the blood vessels of the *heart* and is often used interchangeably with coronary artery disease, or ischemic heart disease. It does *not* encompass cerebrovascular disease, or atherosclerotic disease of the limbs or abdomen.

Case-finding means looking out for a particular disease or problem in *all* patients coming to the doctor irrespective of the reason (cf. screening).

Catastrophic reaction is an abnormal emotional response to being asked to complete a task. Minor forms include truculence, irritability or reluctance to comply. More severe forms may include agitation and crying, and either aggression or absolute refusal to continue.

Cerebral embolism is embolism of thrombotic material to the brain from *any* proximal site, not just the heart (e.g. from atheromatous arteries).

Cerebral infarction means literally death of cerebral tissue and is used for a stroke due to occlusion of either cerebral arteries or veins. It cannot be reliably differentiated from primary intracerebral haemorrhage during life without CT scanning within days or a few weeks of the onset.

Cerebrovascular disease is any disorder affecting the blood vessels of the brain.

Crude incidence (see incidence).

Depressive illness is a morbid state characterized by persistently lowered mood, biological symptoms (e.g. anorexia, insomnia), and pessimistic thoughts about many different aspects of life. There may rarely be delusions or hallucinations.

Disability is the loss of ability to do something. It must be distinguished from handicap (see below).

Drop attacks are sudden falls to the ground with normal, or very brief loss of, consciousness; they may have several causes, and are therefore a symptom not a disease.

Dysarthria is difficulty in speaking due to a problem with articulation.

Dysphagia is difficulty in swallowing.

Dysphasia is used interchangeably with aphasia.

Emotional lability is a disorder of emotional expression in which weeping is provoked by trivial remarks or experiences. Unusual varieties include contextually inappropriate crying (forced weeping) and pathological laughter.

Focal neurological features are features which indicate a focal problem in the brain, e.g. hemiparesis, aphasia (cf. non-focal features).

Handicap is due to disability but varies, even given the same level of disability, because it depends on the patient's ability to cope, or be helped with his particular disability.

Homonymous hemianopia is a visual field defect such that the temporal visual field is lost in one eye along with the nasal visual field in the other.

Hydrocephalus is enlargement of one or more of the ventricles of the brain either because of obstruction of CSF flow, or loss of brain substance.

Inattention, either to sensory or visual stimuli, is the inability to perceive a stimulus on one side of the body when stimuli are applied simultaneously to both sides. The responsible lesion is usually in the contralateral parietal or occipital lobe respectively.

Incidence is the number of new cases in a given population in a given time period, usually 1 year. A crude incidence rate is the overall rate in the population being tested irrespective of age. Age-specific incidence means that the incidence is given separately for particular age bands, and age-adjustment or standardization means that the incidence is calculated for the whole of a given population adjusting its age structure to some standard population such as England and Wales.

Indifference reaction is a state of inappropriate apathy, or indifference to environmental stimulation. It is differentiated from the catastrophic reaction (see above) by the absence of apparent distress.

Intracranial haemorrhage is bleeding within the skull which may be primarily intracerebral or subarachnoid or both.

Lacunar stroke is a particular type of cerebral infarction due to a small infarct deep in the region of the internal capsule, basal ganglia, or brainstem.

Neglect is the same as inattention.

Non-focal neurological features are features which suggest a global reduction in brain function, e.g. faintness, generalized weakness, loss of consciousness (cf. focal neurological features).

Pathological emotionalism (see emotional lability).

Prevalence is the frequency of a given disease in a population of a given size at one particular time. Crude, age-specific and age-adjusted rates can be used (see incidence).

Primary intracerebral haemorrhage is a stroke due to bleeding primarily into the brain substance. During life this can only be reliably differentiated from cerebral infarction by a CT scan within days, or 1 or 2 weeks of the onset.

Primary prevention is reducing the risk of, preventing, or delaying a particular disease when there has been no previous manifestation of that disease (cf. secondary prevention).

Pseudo-dementia is a reversible state of cognitive impairment with defective memory and orientation as well as motor slowing, withdrawal and self-neglect. It is one presentation of depressive illness in the elderly.

Relative risk (see risk).

Reversible ischaemic neurological deficit (RIND) is a term sometimes used for a focal ischaemic episode in the brain which takes more than 24 hours to recover (see transient ischaemic attacks) but which does eventually recover leaving no symptoms or disability.

Risk: Relative risk is the ratio of the incidence of a disease in a population with a given risk factor (e.g. smokers) compared with the incidence in a similar population but without the risk factor (e.g. non-smokers). **Absolute** risk is the risk that a population with a given factor will develop a particular disease. **Attributable** risk is the fraction of a population with a given disease for which a particular risk factor is thought to be responsible.

Risk factor is a variable (e.g. blood pressure) in a population associated with a particular disease, usually positively rather than negatively.

Screening is deliberately setting out to look for a particular disease or risk factor in a population by calling in for examination everyone who is thought to be at risk (cf. case-finding).

Secondary prevention is reducing the risk of, preventing, or delaying the recurrence of a particular disease after it has become clinically manifest (cf. primary prevention).

Stroke is a rapidly developing focal, or at times global (applied to patients with subarachnoid haemorrhage or in coma), deterioration in neurological function when there is no likely cause other than a vascular one, and which causes symptoms for more than 24 hours, or leads to death. It includes cerebral infarction, primary intracerebral haemorrhage, and subarachnoid haemorrhage.

Subarachnoid haemorrhage is a stroke due to spontaneous bleeding primarily onto the surface of the brain within the subarachnoid space.

Subclavian steal causes the symptoms of brainstem ischaemia during arm exercise as a result of reversed flow down the vertebral artery distal to subclavian stenosis or occlusion.

Transient global amnesia is the syndrome, with several causes, of severe global amnesia lasting a few hours but with no loss of personal identity or any other clinical features.

Transient ischaemic attack is an acute loss of brain or eye function with symptoms lasting less than 24 hours and which, after adequate investigation, is presumed to be due to a vascular cause; thrombosis or embolism in the arterial supply to the brain or eye.

APPENDIX 2

This appendix lists scales which we use in both stroke research and care. They are simple, reasonably well validated, and seem to work well.

MODIFIED RANKIN SCORE

0 = No symptoms
1 = Minor symptoms which don't interfere with the lifestyle of the patient
2 = Minor handicap – symptoms which lead to some restriction of lifestyle, but don't interfere with the patients' capacity to look after themselves
3 = Moderate handicap – symptoms which significantly restrict lifestyle and/or prevent totally independent existence.
4 = Moderately severe handicap – symptoms which clearly prevent independent existence though the patient does not need constant attention
5 = Severe handicap – totally dependent existence, requiring constant attention day and night
6 = Dead

This is a very useful and simple system for scoring handicap. It should be explicit whether it is used to score the *whole* patient, or just the stroke. For example, difficulty walking may be due to just a stroke, or to many other factors (arthritis, angina, claudication, etc.) so it should be made absolutely clear how the scale is being used.

BARTHEL SCORE

Function

1. Feeding
   2 = Independent
   1 = Needs some help
   0 = Needs to be fed
2. Bathing
   1 = Able to wash all over
   0 = Needs help
3. Grooming
   1 = Totally independent
   0 = Dependent in some way
4. Dressing
   2 = Independent (no aids)
   1 = Needs help with some items
   0 = Unable to do without help
5. Bowels
   2 = No accidents
   1 = Occasional accidents/help with enema
   0 = Incontinent
6. Bladder
   2 = No accidents
   1 = Occasional incontinence or device used
   0 = Incontinent
7. Toilet
   2 = Independent
   1 = Minor assistance
   0 = Unable to use
8. Transfer (bed to chair)
   3 = Totally independent
   2 = Minimal help needed
   1 = Sit unaided, major help for transfer
   0 = Unable
9. Ambulation
   3 = Independent for 50 metres
   2 = Walk 50 metres with help
   1 = Independent in wheelchair for 50 metres
   0 = Immobile

10. Stairs   2 = Independent
                    1 = Needs physical/verbal support
                    0 = Unable

Barthel score = total of above

This should be scored on the basis of what the patient actually does, *not* what he ought to be able to do. It measures ability in 10 activities, and although often the total score is quoted it is probably better to consider each domain separately.

MINI MENTAL STATE

Introduction

I would like to ask you some questions which we use routinely with everybody. Some of them may seem very simple, and some may seem very difficult, but I hope you won't let yourself be worried or offended by any of them. I would be grateful if you would have a try at all of the questions that I am going to ask you.

Orientation

			Score	Points
1.	What is the:	year	—	1
		season	—	1
		date	—	1
		day	—	1
		month	—	1
2.	Where are we:	country	—	1
		county	—	1
		town or village	—	1
		hospital or street (if at home)	—	1
		ward/house name or number	—	1

Registration
3. Name three objects, taking one second to say each. Then ask the patient all three after you have said them. (Give one point for each correct answer.) Now repeat the answers until patient learns all three.   —   3

Attention and calculation
4. Spell WORLD backwards. (Give one point for each letter in its correct position.) (Serial Sevens is now omitted.)   —   5

Recall
5. Ask for names of three objects learned in Q.3. (Give one point for each correct answer.)   —   3

Language
6. Point to a pencil and a watch. Have the patient name them as you point.   —   2
7. Have the patient repeat 'No ifs ands or buts'   —   1
8. Have the patient follow a three-stage command. (The command must be given with all three parts together.) 'Take this paper in your right hand. Fold the paper in half. Put the paper on the floor.'   .   —   3
9. Have the patient read and obey the following: 'CLOSE YOUR EYES' (write in large letters).   —   1
10. Have the patient write a sentence of his or her choice. (The sentence should contain a subject and an object, and should make sense. Ignore spelling errors when scoring.)   —   1

11. Enlarge the pattern printed below to 1.5 cm per side and have the patient copy it. (Give one point if all sides and angles are preserved and if the intersecting sides form a quadrangle).   —   1

= Total 30

Were any of the following a problem during interview (tick if a problem):

Willingness to co-operate   Hearing
Comprehension of language   Eyesight
Use of language   Dexterity
Literacy

APPENDIX 3

SOURCES OF INFORMATION FOR PATIENTS, PROFESSIONALS, AND CARERS

Books for the patient and family:

Stroke: a practical guide towards recovery R. Langton Hewer and D. T. Wade
Martin Dunitz, London, 1986

Stroke; the facts F. C. Rose and R. Capildeo
Oxford University Press, Oxford, 1981

Caring for the Sick St John Ambulance Association, St Andrew's Ambulance Association, and British Red Cross Society
Dorling Kindersley, London, 1983

A Stroke in the Family Valerie Eaton Griffith
Penguin Books, 1970
The story of Patricia Neal

When Half is Whole: my recovery from stroke Lorna Hewson
Dove Communications, Blackburn, Australia
A well-written book describing the effects of stroke upon the author (an occupational therapist) and her recovery

Living After a Stroke Diana Law and Barbara Paterson
Souvenir Press (Educational and Academic) Ltd, London,
1980
Biography of Diana Law and her recovery from stroke

Sources of information for professional staff

Directory for Disabled People: A handbook of information and opportunities for disabled and handicapped people
Compiled by Ann Darnbrough and Derek Kinrade
Woodhead-Faulkner Ltd, Fitzwilliam House, 32 Trumpington Street, Cambridge CB2 1QY
In association with The Royal Association for Disability and Rehabilitation.
Fourth edition, 1985
This book gives a wide range of practical information concerning many areas such as rights to social security funds, aids, mobility, leisure and holidays. It includes titles of other useful books on, for example, sexual problems.

The Source Book for the Disabled Edited by Glorya Hale
Paddington Press Ltd, London and New York, 1979
A book giving much useful advice on adapting to disability, with many illustrations. Covers many disabilities; not specific to stroke. Includes a section on 'resources' such as addresses of organizations.

Someone To Talk To Directory Routledge and Kegan Paul Ltd, in association with the Mental Health Foundation
This book gives details about 10 000 national and local self-help and community support agencies and organizations for disabled people in Britain and Eire.

Useful addresses

The Chest, Heart and Stroke Association
Tavistock House North
Tavistock Square
London WC1H 9JE
Tel: (01) 387–3012
This association supports people with stroke in many ways:
(a) Producing publications, some free, such as *Stroke – Twenty Questions – and the Answers* and *Understanding Stroke*
(b) Keeping a directory of stroke clubs throughout Britain
(c) Sponsoring many local support groups

Disabled Living Foundation
380–384 Harrow Road
London W9 2HU
Provides a general information service on the non-medical aspects of disability, with expertise on practical problems like aids and adaptations.

Association of Carers
Medway Homes
Balfour Road
Rochester, Kent ME4 6QU
A recently established national organization acting both as a pressure group and a source of information to local support groups

The Red Cross will often loan aids

Often local charities such as the Lions, Round Table, etc, have loan schemes

APPENDIX 4

FURTHER READING

Allen, C. M. C. (1984) The Clinical Diagnosis of Acute Stroke: a review. *Journal of the Royal Society of Medicine*, **77**, 878–81

Binder, L. M. (1984) Emotional problems after stroke. *Stroke*, **15**, 174–7

Coope, J. (1985) Care of hypertensive patients. *GP Update*, **32**, 303–12

Goodstein, R. K. (1983) Overview: cerebrovascular accident and the hospitalised elderly – a multidimensional problem. *American Journal of Psychiatry*, **140**, 141–147

Harrison, M. J. G. and Dyken, M. (1983) *Cerebral Vascular Disease*. London: Butterworths

Lancet Editorial (1985) Treatment of hypertension: the 1985 results. *Lancet*, **2**, 645–6

Rose, G. (1981) Strategy for prevention: lessons from cardiovascular disease. *British Medical Journal*, **282**, 1847–51

Ruskin, A. P. (1983) Understanding stroke and its rehabilitation. *Stroke*, **14**, 438–42

Russell, R. W. (1983) *Vascular Disease of the Central Nervous System*. Edinburgh: Churchill Livingstone

Sandercock, P. and Warlow, C. (1985) Prevention of stroke in the elderly. In: Gray, J. A. M. (ed.) *Prevention of Disease in the Elderly*. Edinburgh: Churchill Livingstone

Wade, D. T., Langton Hewer, R., Skilbeck, C. E. and David, R. M. (1985) *Stroke: A Critical Approach to Diagnosis, Treatment and Management*. London: Chapman & Hall Medical

Warlow, C. P. and Morris, P. (1982) *Transient Ischaemic Attacks*. New York, Marcel Dekker

Warlow, C. P. (1985) Carotid endarterectomy: does it work? *Stroke*, **15,** 1068–76

Warlow, C. P. (1986) Transient ischaemic attacks. In: Trigger, D. R. (ed.) *Advanced Medicine*, 22. London: Baillière Tindall

INDEX